The Natural History Of Iceland

THE

NATURAL HISTORY

OF

ICELAND:

CONTAINING

A particular and accurate Account of the different Soils, burning Mountains, Minerals, Vegetables, Metals, Stones, Beafts, Birds, and Fifhes;
together with the Difpofition, Cuftoms, and Manner of Living of
the Inhabitants. Interfperfed with an Account of the Ifland, by
Mr. Anderson, late Burgo-mafter of Hamburgh.

To which is added,

A METEOROLOGICAL TABLE, with REMARKS.

Tranflated from the Danish Original of

Mr. N. HORREBOW.

And illuftrated with a New General Map of the Ifland.

LONDON:

Printed for A. Linde in Catherine-Street, D. Wilson, and T. Durham in the Strand,
G. Keith in Grace-church-ftreet, P. Davey and B. Law in Ave-mary-lane,
T. Field in Cheapfide, C. Henderson at the Royal-Exchange, and J. Staples in
Stationers-court.

MDCCLVIII.

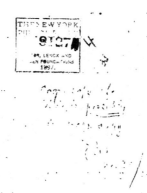

THE

PREFACE.

ICELAND is next to Great-Britain, the largest island in
Europe, and in my humble opinion, deserves in a great measure to be rescued from the obscurity in which it has long drooped;
so much the more, as there is scarce a country the world has
less knowledge, or has conceived a less genuine idea of, chiefly
by reason of the accounts published of it, which are far from
being true, or to be depended upon. The Icelanders themselves
have been as careful as any people on the globe, in noting down
in a simple, plain and honest manner, all the remarkable occur-
rences that have happened in the island since its first discovery,
and their first settling in it; the former of which is supposed to
be in the year 861, and the latter in 874. It were to be wished,
that from their accounts any one had compiled a history of Iceland; as such, no doubt, would convey a true idea of *à nas-
cente republicâ :* but however careful they were in collecting, it
must be said, that they have been somewhat remiss in satisfying
the public with an accurate description of their country ; for the
small treatises of Arngrimo Jonæ, and Theodoro Thorlacio, which
are conducted in the disputative form of controversy, cannot be
looked upon as complete performances, though prettily written.
This work is therefore likely to be left for foreigners, though the
natives are certainly best qualified for it: and indeed, it can be
no easy task for a foreigner, if we consider the extent of the
country, and the many strange phenomena it contains, which make
it almost impossible for him to execute the same properly, unless by
living there a considerable time, he has made himself master of
the language, and informed himself faithfully of every particular. Notwithstanding these difficulties, strangers and foreigners

have

have thought themfelves qualified to give a defcription of this ifland; fome who had only been a fhort time in the ifland, having clapt together a hiftory in a hurry; and others who had never feen the place, having collected all the accounts they could receive from travellers, upon which they founded their hiftory.

Of the firft fort is the famous Blefkenius, who lay a little while on the coaft in a Dutch fhip, was two or three times afhore, and hardly underftood any thing of the language. This gentleman after his return, publifhed a fmall treatife on Iceland, or rather a falfe and fcandalous libel, which was refuted in another fmall treatife publifhed by Arngrimo Jonæ, and intitled *Anatome Blefkeniana*.

Of the fecond fort is the learned Mr. John Anderfon, formerly firft burgo-mafter in Hamburg, who, as he himfelf acknowledges in his preface, had compiled his hiftory from accounts of mafters of fhips, fuper-cargoes, factors, &c. who traded there, and whom he invited to his houfe from Gluckftad, and by interrogating them, and fhewing them his collection of natural curiofities, induced them to give him, as he imagined, a faithful and circumftantial account of all they knew, either by experience or hearfay, relatively to the natural, political, or commercial ftate of Iceland, together with the various occupations and manner of life of the inhabitants. Thus it was, that all he could difcover of them, or otherwife have as a piece of intelligence to be depended upon, he has thrown together, in a crude, indigefted treatife, and fo tranfmitted it to the public. Hence we may fee the foundation his performance leans upon, and to fhew, that the deceafed good gentleman, did not intend to prefent the public with any thing that fhould convey a difadvantagious or falfe idea of the ifland, he afferts, that what he writes is true. As a fenfible and curious man, he had a ftrong defire, and gave himfelf a great deal of trouble to learn fomething more new and more important, as alfo more complete and better grounded, concerning this great, and for many reafons, remarkable ifland, in lieu of the old and imperfect accounts then extant, which abound with romantic tales

and

and falfities, as he declares in his preface : but as he unwittily
addreffed himfelf to very improper perfons, in order to acquire
the defired intelligence of that ifland, the old falfe accounts and
romantic tales, ftill fubfift with their additions, the author's
good intention is fruftrated, and the public deceived.

Mafters of fhips, fuper-cargoes, and the like, from whom
the late burgo-mafter Anderfon had his whole account, cannot
be deemed competent judges in this refpect, though even fome
of them fhould be allowed underftanding enough to examine
into the natural and political ftate of the country. It is natural to think, that their employments deprive them of the opportunity of coming at any intelligence to be depended upon :
for they lie in a harbour in one corner or other of the ifland, and
are fo bufy all the while, fome with merchandizing, and others
with loading and unloading their fhips, that they have little or
no leifure time to examine into the nature and conftitution of
the country, much lefs into the occupations of the inhabitants,
who while the company's fhips lie there, have nothing to do but
to take care of their hay and harveft : they do not fifh much at
that time, becaufe they cannot fo well dry the fifh : and fome
of them are a good deal employed in trading with the merchants, and keep conftantly at the factories. If then thefe
mafters of fhips and others, cannot judge properly of the conftitution of the country, by a better reafon they may be thought
little converfant with the air of the climate, and the degrees of
heat and cold, fo much the more, as thofe that trade to Gluckftad are there only in the fummer. Thofe who gave an account that it was fo hot, that they were obliged to go almoft
naked, had that day, I fuppofe, great quantities of fifh to weigh
off, and fend aboard their refpective fhips. On the other hand,
perhaps fome of them being obliged by fome accident happening to the fhip, to winter there againft their will, became fo
unhappy, and out of humour, that all things feemed bad to
them; or much worfe than they really were, and confequently
deprived them of all inclination to bring matters to an impar-
tial fcrutiny. Hence may be derived the accounts of long perpetual piercing colds, &c. whereas neither heat nor cold can be

deter-

determined fo well by external fenfation, as by thermomical obfervations, the only proper teft in this refpect.

These reafons may evince the extent of their experience, or
rather how very flight it was, which, no doubt, they difplay-
ed in glaring colours, when they had the honour to be invited
and received fo politely by the firft burgo-mafter of the great
city of Hamburg. They thought it incumbent on them at
leaft, to inform this learned gentleman, of all that he feemed
defirous to know, and they would not appear fo fimple or de-
void of curiofity, as not to give fome account of every particular in the ifland, which perhaps they made feveral voyages
to, and confequently full of their own knowledge and experience, could not help telling fome things they knew, and others
they knew nothing of.

In this manner the late burgo-mafter Anderfon's credulity
has been impofed upon, not doubting, but all thefe accounts
were authentic and inconteftable, as being received from perfons who vifited the ifland every year, and had collected all
their intelligence at firft hand, and from their own knowledge
and experience. As he alfo knew, that the public had little or
no knowledge of this remote country, he was willing to oblige
them in fome meafure, by giving his manufcript to be perufed
by every one that defired it, and his upright and laudable in-
tentions were at laft fully completed by his heirs printing and
publifhing the fame.

This work, afterwards tranflated from the High-Dutch into
the Danifh language, was well received and read in both, with
a great deal of pleafure, and befides, was believed to be a perfect illuftration or genuine account of that country. Though
it muft be allowed, that it abounds with many pretty and ingenious notes and remarks, anfwerable to the character of fo learned and admirable an author, yet it is certain, that the facts on
which it is grounded, are for the greater part falfe, and expofe
the ignorance, the miftaken ideas, and withal the bad difpofi-
tions of the hearts of thofe againft the Icelanders, who foifted
fuch fpurious accounts upon the late Mr. Anderfon's credulity.

To

To undeceive the public, and make void the severe and false
accusations contained in that book against this island, I have
made it my business to publish this treatise, which contains a
very faithful account of the island, the air, the people, and
their various occupations. In order to this, I have followed
Mr. Anderson, article by article, declaring what is false in each,
relating what is true and matter of fact, and introducing a variety of new things, of which he has taken no manner of notice.
As his account of Iceland is entirely false, and conveys a wrong
idea of the country, and every thing belonging to it, it was
highly necessary that the public should have the affair cleared
up, and placed in a true light, notwithstanding the name of
this learned and admirable man, which gives such a sanction to
his book, that scarce any doubt of the truth of the facts alledged in it; though I dare say, that had that worthy man
known how he had been abused, he never would have suffered
it to appear.

Of a different nature is this treatise which I here give to the
public concerning Iceland. It is founded upon what I myself
have seen and experienced, during the two years I lived in the
island: the historical part of the events that happened before my
arriving there, I received from worthy and learned people in the
country, who have been eye-witnesses themselves of them, and
were capable of giving better accounts than the common people,
from whom the masters of ships or super-cargoes, had their
intelligence. I made several observations with an excellent Paris
quadrant, and ascertained the elevation of the pole, by means
of a lunar eclipse, which happened December 1750. By a
telescope accurately furnished with a micrometer, I took the
exact latitude of the island, and having determined it in a nicer
manner than it ever was before, found that Iceland lies almost four
degrees more to the east than it has hitherto been computed.

On the barometer and thermometer, I made observations during two years, by which the weight of the atmosphere, and
the degrees of heat and cold, were discovered, and found to be
quite the reverse of what was imagined. In short, I had the
happiness to make such meteorological and physical observations,

tions, in regard to the air and earth, that many things are now brought to light, which before were either buried in obscurity, or hinted at in a confused and imperfect manner.

Such is this treatise, I now have the honour to lay before the public. It is not to be considered as a complete description of the island, which none can be capable of effecting, unless they have lived there a considerable time, are versed in the necessary sciences, and have a sufficient support; but it contains such an account of the country, as is litterally true, and may be depended upon, and which at present the public may be satisfied with, till that performance appears to answer the pompous title taken notice of in the * journal of the *literati*, which I sincerely wish any one was capable of executing.

As this treatise therefore is of a different complexion to any other hitherto published, so also is the annexed map. All others of this kind are far from being exact, more especially that published with Mr. Anderson's treatise. As to the annexed, it was carefully copied and taken from a large original map of Iceland, the work of some years, and done by some of the officers of his Majesty's corps of engineers, who were sent for this purpose to Iceland. In 1734, it was completed by captain Knopff, and by his Majesty's gracious command, delivered to me, that I might publish a copy of it with this history. This map, which was never before published, is the exactest of any extant of Iceland, and I do not doubt but that the public will receive it with a great deal of pleasure and satisfaction.

A few remarks have been made upon the map by way of introduction to the treatise, and to render it more plain and distinct.

The meteorological observations which I made during my two years stay there, are printed at the end of the treatise, with remarks and explanations, how they were performed.

* A periodical or public paper so called.

Remarks

Remarks on the map.

I before obferved, that the annexed map was the work of fome of his Majefty's engineers, and completed by captain Knopff. No alteration is made in it, except the placing of Beffefted according to my obfervations in Iceland, in its true latitude and longitude, and confequently afcertaining the fituation of the whole ifland, by removing it four degrees more to the eaft, than has hitherto been known.

The phyfical length of Iceland, as I have fet it down in the treatife, is about feven hundred and twenty miles, but in this map it appears to be fomething lefs. However, none I fuppofe, are able to determine which is the jufter. My calculation, in regard to the length of the ifland, is founded partly upon fome ancient Icelandifh writers, and partly upon the reckonings of the inhabitants, according to their Thing-manna-leid, which is a certain length of ground that a man travels each day when he is on a journey to the affizes. Thefe are not a certain number of meafured miles; but a Thing-manna-leid, according to the acceptation of the word, makes fometimes thirty, and fometimes forty-eight Englifh miles, and in confequence of this way of meafuring, they make the ifland one hundred and twenty Danifh, or feven hundred and twenty Englifh miles long.

The map is divided into four quarters, as eaft, fouth, weft and north, which are marked with double dots, in contradiftinction to the divifions with fingle ones, which are the fyffels, or certain diftricts under a fyffelman or tax-gatherer, who is a juftice of the peace.

The names of the harbours and principal places, to make them more intelligible, I have put in the Danifh language, but fuch as are eafy to underftand, I have left as they were, as thingey, eyefiord, ey fignifying an ifland.

In order that any place may be found out expeditioufly in the map, I have drawn angles through the degrees, which are lettered at the top and bottom, and figures in roman characters on the fides, and have made an alphabetical table of the names

b of

T H E P R E F A C E.

of all the places on the map, with the letters and numbers prefixed, to fhew where each place lies, which table for explanation fake is bound up with it.

An ALPHABETICAL TABLE
Of the names of the places on the map.

The letters ftand at top and bottom, the numbers on the fides, and the place fought in the angle on the map.

A.

Akur ey   C. III. —

Vide the printed table for the reft.

T H E

THE

CONTENTS.

CHAPTER I.

ICELAND, its fituation and extent. Page 1

CHAP. II.

Concerning the earth and the different foils. 2

CHAP. III.

The manner of travelling in this country. 4

CHAP. IV.

In what manner it is inhabited. 5

CHAP. V.

Concerning earthquakes in this ifland. 7

CHAP. VI.

Concerning fiery eruptions and volcanos in the earth. 8

CHAP. VII.

Concerning the burning mountains. 11

CHAP. VIII.

Concerning the mountain Hecla. 15

CHAP. IX.

A brief and general defcription of Iceland with regard to its fize, and the peculiar properties of the earth and mountains.
page 17

CHAP. X.

Concerning a lake which takes fire three times a year. 19

CHAP. XI.

Concerning the hot waters. 20

CHAP. XII.

Concerning the property and quality of the rocks and mountains, in which probably marble may be found. 25

CHAP. XIII.

Concerning cryftals. 26

CHAP. XIV.

Concerning pumice ftone. ibid.

CHAP. XV.

Concerning the metallic ores found in this country. ibid.

CHAP. XVI.

Concerning rofin and turf. 27

CHAP. XVII.

Concerning agates. 28

CHAP. XVIII.

Concerning fulphur. ibid.

CHAP. XIX.

Concerning falt, whether any be found in Iceland. 31

CHAP.

CHAP. XX.

Concerning forests and trees.   page 32

CHAP. XXI.

Concerning the pasture-land and grass.   34

CHAP. XXII.

Whether there are wholsome herbs and roots in this island.   35

CHAP. XXIII.

Concerning the fruits of the earth.   36

CHAP. XXIV.

Concerning the cultivating of the land.   38

CHAP. XXV.

Concerning sea-weeds, and vegetables of the ocean.   41

CHAP. XXVI.

Whether there are wild beasts in this island.   42

CHAP. XXVII.

Concerning the fox.   43

CHAP. XXVIII.

Concerning horses.   44

CHAP. XXIX.

Concerning the sheep.   45

CHAP. XXX.

Concerning goats.   51

CHAP. XXXI.

Concerning cows and bullocks.   52

ç   CHAP.

THE CONTENTS.

CHAP. XXXII.

Concerning their milk, curds and whey. page 53

CHAP. XXXIII.

Concerning butter and cheese. ibid.

CHAP. XXXIV.

The manner of slaughtering their cattle, and curing the meat. 54

CHAP. XXXV.

Concerning their hogs. 55

CHAP. XXXVI.

Concerning tame fowl. 56

CHAP. XXXVII.

Concerning wild land-fowl. ibid.

CHAP. XXXVIII.

Concerning birds of prey. 57

CHAP. XXXIX.

Concerning the eagle. ibid.

CHAP. XL.

Concerning the hawk. 58

CHAP. XLI.

Concerning the falcon. ibid.

CHAP. XLII.

Concerning owls. 61

CHAP. XLIII.

Concerning ravens. ibid.

CHAP.

CHAP. XLIV.

Concerning the shore, or coast-birds.   page 61

CHAP. XLV.

Concerning the shore-birds that are fit to eat.   63

CHAP. XLVI.

Concerning the wild geese.   64

CHAP. XLVII.

Concerning wild ducks, and down-birds.   Ibid.

CHAP. XLVIII.

Concerning the diver or the plungeon.   67

CHAP. XLIX.

Concerning the lomen, or northern diver.   ibid.

CHAP. L.

Concerning the geir or vulture.   68

CHAP. LI.

Concerning the shore-birds nests.   ibid.

CHAP. LII.

Concerning the shore-birds eggs.   69

CHAP. LIII.

Concerning the vast quantity of shore-fish.   70

CHAP. LIV.

Concerning the shore-fish, or such as in general keep along the
coast.   71

CHAP. LV.

Concerning herrings.   ibid.

CHAP.

C H A P.   LVI.

Concerning the cod.   page 73

C H A P.   LVII.

Concerning the ling.   80

C H A P.   LVIII.

Concerning the haddock.   81

C H A P.   LIX.

Concerning the whiting.   ibid.

C H A P.   LX.

Concerning the fort of cod which the Icelanders call tifling.   82

C H A P.   LXI.

Concerning the cole-fifh.   ibid.

C H A P.   LXII.

Concerning flounders.   83

C H A P.   LXIII.

Concerning the turbot.   ibid.

C H A P.   LXIV.

Concerning mackarel.   ibid.

C H A P.   LXV.

Concerning the whale.   85

C H A P.   LXVI.

Concerning the porpus.   86

C H A P.   LXVII.

Concerning the fea-calf.   87

C H A P.

CHAP. LXVIII.

Concerning the fword-fifh, or faw-fifh.   page 88

CHAP. LXIX.

Concerning fea-bulls, and fea-cows.   ibid.

CHAP. LXX.

Concerning the feal.   ibid.

CHAP. LXXI.

Concerning frefh water fifh.   89

CHAP. LXXII.

Concerning fnakes.   91

CHAP. LXXIII.

Concerning infects and vermin.   ibid.

CHAP. LXXIV.

Concerning mice.   92

CHAP. LXXV.

Concerning the fun when above and below the horizon.   ibid.

CHAP. LXXVI.

Concerning the *aurora borealis*, or north light.   94

CHAP. LXXVII.

Concerning thunder and meteors.   95

CHAP. LXXVIII.

Concerning parhelions, or mock funs.   96

CHAP. LXXIX.

Concerning the feafons of the year.   97

CHAP. LXXX.

Concerning the weather.   99

d   CHAP.

CHAP. LXXXI.

Concerning the ebb and flood, or the tides.   page 100

CHAP. LXXXII.

Concerning the fea water.   101

CHAP. LXXXIII.

Concerning the climate of Iceland, and the conftitution of the inhabitants.   102

CHAP. LXXXIV.

Concerning the prevailing difeafes in Iceland.   105

CHAP. LXXXV.

How they bring up their children.   106

CHAP. LXXXVI.

Concerning their manner of dreffing victuals.   107

CHAP. LXXXVII.

Concerning the fcarcity of bread.   110

CHAP. LXXXVIII.

Concerning their drink.   111

CHAP. LXXXIX.

Concerning their drefs.   113

CHAP. XC.

Concerning their habitations.   116

CHAP. XCI.

Concerning their genius, and natural difpofition of mind.   119

CHAP. XCII.

Whether they delight in learning any thing.   120

CHAP.

C H A P. XCIII.

Concerning their occupations. page 122

C H A P. XCIV.

Concerning their cattle-trade. 123

C H A P. XCV.

Concerning the Icelanders tannery. ibid.

C H A P. XCVI.

Concerning some other of their employments. 124

C H A P. XCVII.

Concerning their manner of merchandizing. 126

C H A P. XCVIII.

Concerning accompts and payments. 127

C H A P. XCIX.

Concerning the goods they export. 128

C H A P. C.

Concerning the goods they import. ibid.

C H A P. CI.

Concerning their weights and measures. 129

C H A P. CII.

Concerning their religion. 130

C H A P. CIII.

Concerning the ecclesiastical state of this island. ibid.

C H A P. CIV.

Concerning their churches. 132

C H A P. CV.

Concerning the clergy. 135

CHAP. CVI.

Concerning the education of their children.   page 136

CHAP. CVII.

Concerning the vices of the Icelanders.   137

CHAP. CVIII.

Concerning their nuptial ceremonies.   138

CHAP. CIX.

Whether the Icelanders are fond of the game of chefs.   139

CHAP. CX.

Concerning their manner of dancing.   ibid.

CHAP. CXI.

Concerning their civil government.   140

CHAP. CXII.

Concerning the reft of his Majefty's fervants or officers in the ifland.   ibid.

CHAP. CXIII.

Concerning their laws.   142

CHAP. CXIV.

Concerning executions, or punifhments by death.   144

CHAP. CXV.

Conclufion.   ibid.

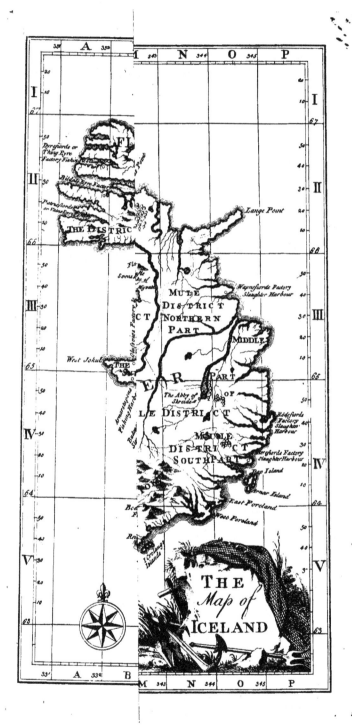

THE
Map of
ICELAND

THE

NATURAL HISTORY

OF

ICELAND.

CHAPTER I.

Its Situation and Extent.

CELAND is an island in the Atlantic ocean, which, by the nicest observations I could make with a very good French quadrant, from a seat of his Danish majesty, situate in the south part of this island, and called Beſſeſted; lies 64 deg. 4 min. north latitude. By a lunar eclipse I took the longitude, which from the meridian of London is 25 degrees west, being 4 degrees more to the east than it has hitherto been computed. This discovery, I hope, will be of use to those that navigate these seas. To be particular in the length and breadth would be a very difficult matter, by reason of its requiring very long and tedious journies to make the necessary observations. The length from east to west may be computed at 120 Danish or 720 English miles, and the breadth in the narrowest parts at 41 Danish or 246 English, though in most parts from north to south it is 60 Danish or 360 English. Thus the breadth may safely be reckoned at 50 Danish or 300 English miles. This calculation, I am certain, is very moderate. Mr. Anderson, late burgo-master of Hamburg, wrote and published some time ago an account of this island with a map an-

B   nexed

nexed to it, which takes in 11 degrees in length and 3 and a half in breadth *.

CHAP. II.

Concerning the Earth and the different Soils.

VERY probable it is, that this island has undergone a confiderable change by the univerfal deluge, as well as many other places : for it is an uneven country covered with rocks and rugged mountains, much like Norway and a great part of Italy †. The Alps and Pyrenean mountains make on the Italian borders a great tract of land. In Europe we find many countries, whofe face appears as irregular as Iceland, with vaft mountains and valleys. The coaft is not crowded with little iflands and rocks like Norway, but for the better part lies expofed to the ocean. To the fouth, but very few appear; and thefe are called (Fugle Skiarene) or Birds Rocks, becaufe birds breed on them in abundance. At the entrance of fome of the harbours, particularly Oreback, Grindevig and Boefand, are many little rocks and banks in the fea near the coaft, which failors ought to avoid, as alfo in the midft of the entrance into the harbour of Hafnefiorden, otherwife a very fine and fafe harbour ‡.

Some few iflands lying in the fea off the coaft, are very fertile, and bare excellent grafs. They are not inhabited. Moft of them lie weftward from Bredefiord, and extend a little beyond Dalefyffel, in which diftrict are many of fuch valuable and important iflands. Very few appear to the north and fouth; Papoe, I believe, is the only one to the eaft. In the interior parts of the ifland are very extenfive heaths and plains, together with vaft ‖

---

* Mr. Anderfon in his defcription of Iceland publifhed at Hamburg, fays, that the ifland of Iceland lies pretty far up in the north fea, and is generally reckoned feventy Danifh or four hundred and twenty Englifh miles long, and forty-one Danifh or two hundred and forty-fix Englifh broad. This our author, even by Mr. Anderfon's maps, proves to be wrong, as alfo that it does not lie in the north fea, but in the Atlantic ocean, the north fea, as he fays, ending at Hetland.

† Mr. Anderfon calls it an irregular fpot abounding with a multiplicity of barren Mountains.

‡ The fame Author fays the coaft is covered all round with a multitude of broken rocks, or as he calls them (blind) fcarce peeping above the furface of the water.

‖ He alfo alledges that the interior parts of this ifland abound with vaft high rocks and mountains, fhattered and torn from each other; always covered with ice and fnow, and uninhabitable by the human fpecies.

mountains,

mountains, many of which are always covered with ice and fnow. The greater part of them are paffable, and have roads over them, where fome hundreds of horfes and men pafs every year. Moft of the northern people travel acrofs the large chain of rocks that run along the country, and fetch their winter ftock of dried fifh from the fouth and weft parts. The mountains in the common road are not fo difficult to pafs as thofe on the Alps and Pyrenees. On the top of fome of thefe mountains are plains of twenty or twenty-five Englifh miles extent. There are alfo in feveral places large tracts of land with good grafs for pafture, and great lakes abounding with variety of fine fifh, and in fome places fand ground. Some of the mountains, which at all times are covered with ice and fnow, are called Jokeler. From the tops a dark, futty, thick, ftinking water continually flows like a great river. Thefe Jokeler are not the higheft part of the mountains, there being many near them much higher, yet without fnow continually on them. This may probably be owing to the nitrous quality of the earth. There appears a very extraordinary phænomenon in thefe places, which may rather belong to a metaphyfical than hiftorical defcription. However, it will not be amifs to give a brief account of it in the ftrange property of thefe places called Jokells, which increafe in bulk, and again diminifh and change their appearance almoft every day. For inftance, paths are feen in the fand, made by travellers that paffed the day before. When followed, they lead to a place, like a large pond or lake, frozen over, very dangerous to pafs, and not there the day before. This obliges travellers to go two or three Englifh miles round. Then they come again to the very path oppofite to that they were obliged to leave. In a few days the interrupted path appears again, all the ice and water having, as it were, vanifhed. Sometimes travellers are bold enough to venture over the ice rather than go fo much about. But it often happens that their horfes falling into the great breaks which are fometimes in the ice, it is not in their power to fave them. A few days after thefe very horfes are feen lying on the top of the flat ice, where before was a hole feveral fathom deep, but now clofed up and frozen. The ice muft therefore in this intermediate time melt away, and the water freeze again. Hence it may be concluded, that there is

no

no fure road round and over thefe mountains, but by thus continually paffing and repaffing. Sometimes travellers meet with
accidents, but not very often. Thefe kind of Jokells are only in
Skaftefields Syffel, a fouth part of the country. Hecla and the
weftern Jokells are of another kind, and do not change their appearance in this manner. Thefe confift of many ftony rocks and
mountains. Moft of the latter produce fome vegetable.

CHAP. III.

The manner of travelling in this country.

THERE has not been a fiery eruption from any of thefe
mountains, neither has the ground taken fire fince the year
1730. This very feldom happens, and even when it does, it
occupies but a fmall tract at a time. Travellers cannot therefore
be much obftructed by it. The rocks fometimes crack and are
rent afunder here as in all other mountainous places, and by
falling, chance fometimes to cover a good piece of ground, and
bury a hut or farm *. This alfo happens but very feldom. If
in a road, it is foon cleared away and the paffage made free.
They are obliged to tranfport every thing on the backs of horfes.
Carts and waggons are not ufed, though in many places they may.
As an inftance of the goodnefs of fome of the roads, I have
known thofe, that in a fummer's day, from the rifing of the fun,
to the fetting, have rode 120 Englifh miles, and that acrofs the
mountains from north to fouth. The annual circuits of the
judges, their attendants, and baggage are performed on horfe-
back. Some of them from the eaftward make a circuit of upwards of 400 Englifh miles. I only mention thefe particulars to
fhew that the roads are tolerable, and that the inhabitants may
tranfport their goods and wares to and from any part of the
ifland. When the Iceland company's fhips arrive, the people flock
from all parts of the ifland to purchafe their commodities. From
Hoolum upwards of 100 horfes fet out every year for the fouth-

---

* Mr. Anderfon fays that the whole country is overfpread with ftones and broken
rocks; that there is no poffibility of ufing carts or waggons; that the people muft
travel moftly afoot, and that the beft part is hardly fit for a horfe, it being exceffive
dangerous either to climb, ride or walk.

ward

ward to buy up dried fish. Other parts according to their abilities, fend 10, 20 or 30 horfes, for the fame kind of trade.
From the north country they generally carry butter and a quantity of their woollen manufactures to barter them in the fouth
country againft fish, by which means feveral thoufand horfes
annually pass and repafs thefe great mountains *.

C H A P. IV.

In what manner it is inhabited.

THIS ifland is not very populous †, although the natives, as
well as foreigners who fettle among them, feldom leave
the country; and thofe that do, have as ftrong a propenfity to
return as any people whatever to their native place. What
chiefly wafted this country of inhabitants, was a peftilential difeafe
that raged in the fourteenth century, called the ‡ forte död, or
black death. It almoft fwept away every foul from off the
ifland. None fcarce remaining to relate the circumftances of the
dreadful calamity, it was accordingly left out in the annals of
Iceland, where nothing elfe remarkable is omitted. Since its
being firft peopled, thofe that efcaped this great devaftation faved
themfelves by taking refuge in the mountains, and by tradition
relate, that the low and flat country was covered with a thick
fog during the time of this plague. This difeafe extended itfelf
to Norway, Sweden and Denmark and carried off fo many thoufands in thofe countries, that they could not fpare people for this
colony ‖. However the few remaining inhabitants fince increafed
to, I believe, about fourfcore thoufand fouls; which is but a
fmall number for a country of 700 miles extent, and therefore

* Mr. Anderfon fays that none take the trouble of clearing away the broken
rocks and ftone-heaps that fall into the roads; becaufe the inhabitants here, as in
moft barren and defolate mountainous countries, have little or no occafion, much
lefs encouragement to travel.
 † The fame Author is of opinion that the reafon why Iceland is but thinly inhabited, is owing to its being from time to time afflicted with earthquakes and devafta-
tions, which ftill continue.
 ‡ Bifhop Pontoppidan takes notice of this difeafe in his natural hiftory of
Norway.
 ‖ Mr. Anderfon fays the inhabited part of this ifland is chiefly along the coaft, or
at moft not farther than thirty Englifh miles from it, and there only a few fmall
houfes. As for any towns of trade, they are not at all to be met with.

not one tenth part of this ifland is properly inhabited or cultivated. Befides this plague or forte död, feveral other calamities raged at fundry times. In 1697, 1698, and 1699, many died of hunger, and in one only parifh 120. In 1707, the fmall pox carried off upwards of 20,000, and was fucceeded by a fort of plague. The fmall pox is very fatal here. Many other reafons may be added why this place is ufually thin of people : but as this is not owing immediately to any property in the earth or quality in the air, we fhall omit fpeaking farther on this head. The greateft number of the inhabitants live near the fea along the coaft. A great many notwithftanding live fcattered about 100 or 120 Englifh miles from the fea. There are alfo feveral trading towns or fac-tories. At each of the twenty-two harbours of this ifland is a trading town or factory, where the company of merchants trade with the inhabitants. Thefe trading towns are not to be com-pared with places of that denomination in other countries ; for they confift only of three or four dwelling houfes for the merchants of the Iceland company, with a fhop, warehoufe and kitchen. This, which in the main, is no more than a factory, they call a trading town ; the reft of their buildings about the country are fingle houfes or hutts with a yard round about, and a field contiguous which they call (tun). The reft of their land the proprietor lets out fometimes to different people to build on. Thefe proprietors are called Hiauleyemænd : for Hia in the Iceland language is *near*, and imports a people, who have grounds near their houfes. The houfe is called Hiauleye. They are alfo diftinguifhed from thofe that have only hutts, as being poffeffed of ground and grafs to keep a cow or more, which the others have not. This manner takes place over the whole country, fo that no villages are met with. The intire country is divided into parifhes, and each houfe ftands feparate. However, in fome places may be feen 20, 30, and even 50 buildings with their grounds, befides hutts. If thefe can be deemed villages, there are many of the kind in the ifland. This is not the only country inhabited in this manner. The ifland of Bornholm in the Baltic, a fine fpot of ground has not a village in it. In many of the Danifh provinces each farm ftands detached, and I cannot help obferving, that it feems moft convenient for every farm houfe to ftand apart, and to have its

ground

ground contiguous, if for nothing more than to prevent the accidents of fire from fpreading. In mountainous countries it is alfo more rational to build where a fpot of ground is found fit for culture, than to ftand for form and order *. That the inhabitants are more numerous towards the fea-coaft than the interior parts of the country is owing to the fifheries, which yield a better maintenance than the produce of the land, the cultivating of which has not been much attended to fince the dreadful plague.

CHAP. V.

Concerning earthquakes in this ifland.

THERE are but two places where the earth is fulphureous, namely, in the diftrict of Hufevig and to the fouth near Kryfevig. It is true, in fome other parts, where warm baths have been difcovered, the earth retains a kind of fulphureous fmell. The inhabitants informed me that fometimes they had earthquakes, but that they feldom do any great mifchief. During the two years I was there I felt none, though I was once told there had been one. I fuppofe the fhock was but flight †. To the fouthward in Rangervalle and Arnefs parifhes earthquakes are perceived, and fometimes in Guldbringe and the parifhes adjacent; but hardly ever weftward or northward. There have been inftances of houfes fhook down, but the inhabitants ufually fave themfelves. I don't find, that the greateft fhocks they ever had, were ever attended with any eruption of fire or water out of the bowels of the earth. Clefts have been perceived in the rocks and chafms in the earth, and it is very probable that fuch have been occafioned by earthquakes; but from all that I could gather it feems that earthquakes are not there very common; neither do any extraordinary accidents happen by them, if compared with thofe in Italy, Sicily and the American iflands ‡. As

many

---

* Mr. Anderfon fays that the old fafhioned way of building continues to this day, without any regular order.

† The fame Author afferts, that this ifland is but as one rock full of deep holes and caverns, mines, minerals, and burning vapours; therefore the moft likely place in the world for earthquakes. He adds, that they often happen, and fometimes very dreadful.

‡ The fame Author gives the following account of a dreadful earthquake that happened in 1726, at Skageftrand in the north part of this ifland. There was, fays he, a violent

many fabulous ftories have been told about this country and the
dreadful earthquakes which happened in it, I made it my bufinefs to get the beft intelligence I could in this refpect.   In the
year 1720, near Skageftrand in the parifh of Hunnevatn, a rock
of an, enormous fize, probably undermined by length of time
and a continual current of melted fnow from it, fell down upon
a fubterjacent valley, and made a moft horrid noife.   The valley
was remarkable for very fine pafture land; a rivulet ran through
it, and a cottage ftood not far off.   This great rock filled the
valley, crufhed the cottage, and killed every foul in it but one.
The courfe of the water being hereby ftopt, the rivulet overflowed
all the country about, till it rofe fo high as to flow over the rock.
Then it fell into its ufual channel, but on one fide all the
low land is ftill overflowed, not unlike a fpacious lake.   This
heavy fall muft have fhook the earth confiderably all around, and
the perfon that efcaped muft have heard a great noife.   The neighbouring people might very likely take this to be an earthquake, but
it certainly was not.

C H A P. VI.

Concerning fiery eruptions and volcanos in the earth.

I HAVE before obferved. that fulphur is only found in two
parts of the ifland, in the diftrict of Hufevig and Kryfevig.
The laft place affords alfo fome faltpetre.   It were to be wifhed
one could difcover more of it in other parts of the ifland.   Excepting thefe two places, fulphur is fcarce found in any other
part *.   I have even ftood by to have deep holes dug in the earth in
different parts, but never difcovered fulphur or faltpetre any where
elfe.   The turf here has a fulphureous fort of fmell, as it has in
moft countries †.   Here are alfo various forts of earth, clayey,

a violent earthquake in the night time, and a very great rock funk into the earth to
an immenfe depth, which afterwards was filled with water, and became a very fpacious lake.   About the diftance of eight or nine Englifh miles from this place there
ftood a lake, which the neighbouring inhabitants imagined bottomlefs.   This at the
fame inftant became dry, and the bottom thereof rofe up higher than the adjacent land.
* Mr. Anderfon fays that when they have dug five or fix inches deep in the
ground, they find intire lumps of fulphur and a deal of faltpetre, which deftroys
the fertility of the earth.
† This Author alfo alledges, that the earth often takes fire by the fermentation of
various combuftibles, as of iron ore, faltpetre, fulphur, &c.   This fire runs. frequently along the'furface of the earth.   It likewife burns underground, and makes the
earth quite unferviceable.

fandy,

fandy, ftony, and very good mould in many places fit for vegetation when properly cultivated. This I know by experience as
fhall appear in the fequel. In 1728, in the parifh of Norder-
fyffel, fire happening to iffue out of a mountain, fet the fulphureous earth around in flames, melted and made it run like water
to a place called My-vatne, where it flowed into a lake. This
efflux of melted matter can only happen in the two afore-
mentioned places. It has not been heard of from the year
1000 till 1728. In the fouth country it was never heard of,
but in the parifhes of Guldbringe and Arnes, and in thofe of
Hnappedals, Borgefiords and Snefeldsnefs. There are fome flight
accounts of the like in the high mountains between the north
and fouth country. But a few tracts of land, and exceeding
fmall in comparifon to the whole ifland, are thus liable to take
fire. Such grounds as have been burnt in this manner, are called
by the inhabitants Hraun, and moft of them were in the fame
condition they now are when the Norwegians firft began to fettle
here; for the prefent inhabitants can give no account of any
happening from the year 1000 till 1728 *, which I fhall relate
according to the moft authentic accounts I could receive from
very credible and worthy people in the ifland. In the year 1726,
in the parifh of Norderfyffell a few fhocks of an earthquake being
felt, a great mountain called Krafle made a horrid and frightful
rumbling noife, fucceeded by thick fmoke and fire that burft
forth and threw out ftones and afhes in a manner terrible to behold. Two perfons at that inftant happened to be travelling
along the foot of the mountain. The fire rufhed about them ;
they were forely frightened, and every moment expected to be
confumed, but happily efcaped unhurt. It being very calm
weather the afhes and ftones were not carried to any great diftance,
and by this means the adjacent country was not much damaged.
This mountain continued burning for fome time, abating at in-

---

* Mr. Anderfon tells us, that in the year 1729, in the parifh of Huufwich, there
broke out a fire from the earth and deftroyed the little town of Myconfu and all the
neighbouring land. All the churches, houfes, fheep, horfes and horned cattle were
at once confumed to afhes. The flames grazed the furface of the ground with fuch
rapidity that the inhabitants could hardly fave themfelves by the moft precipitate
flight. Six parifhes were in the utmoft danger of being totally deftroyed by the fire ;
but three miraculoufly-efcaped, and the fire, which no human fkill could conquer,
was in a few days extinguifhed by a thick fog and heavy rains.

D   tervals,

tervals, and then breaking out again. No earthquake was perceived, except some slight shocks before the fire began to rage. In the year 1728, from the flames that gushed out, the sulphureous earth in the mountain took fire, burnt for some time, and afterwards became a fluid, running in a slow stream down the south side of the hill, to the low land, as far as a great lake called Myvatne, of thirty-six English miles circumference and eighteen from the mountain. The neighbouring inhabitants being apprehensive of the danger, moved away in the spring of 1729; and the summer following, having stripped their churches and houses of all their timber, brought the same away with them. In the autumn of that year the stream had reached, in the valley or low lands the edge of the lake. It overflowed the three farms of Reikehlid, Groef and Fagreness, and run all over the grounds belonging to them; it also passed round the church, which happily standing on higher ground escaped. At last it took its course into the lake and made a horrible crackling and hissing. It continued still running till the year 1730, and then ceased of itself; probably for want of fuel to keep it alive. This running matter being afterwards congealed, looked like calcined stones. It is called by the natives Hraun. The inhabitants soon rebuilt their huts and churches. Reikehlid, with half its grounds was totally destroyed; but was soon after reinstated on a more convenient spot. As for the other two farms which suffered the same fate, no ground could be found near the place to rebuild them upon. The only damage sustained was in these farms; for not a living creature was hurt. The lake of My-vatne into which this burning matter flowed was filled up at the place where it emptied itself. Before this accident the water was there very deep, and was well stocked with a great many fish, especially small herrings; but for a long time after hardly any were seen: they avoided the place from an aversion to the sulphur, or perhaps died of the stench. At present they are as plenty as ever. This matter as it ran slowly along, appeared like fluid metal and probably consisted of melted brimstone, stones and gravel; but it did not throughout its course set any of the earth on fire. Its flames were confined to the burning rock, which abounded with sulphur. The Icelanders call it the burning stone. This is the truth of what
happened

happened by the mountain of Krafle's taking fire. The fame lafted four years. Since that time no fiery eruption of any kind appeared in the ifland. I fpoke with a perfon who travelled in thofe parts, whilft this ftuff was flowing. He faid that it ran very even and quiet, that he went up to the edge of it, and lighted his pipe by it.

C H A P. VII.

Concerning the burning mountains.

THIS extenfive and mountainous ifland is reported to abound with burning mountains : but from all the accounts I could gather, I do not find twenty all over the ifland that have ever burn'd *. I before obferved, that here are all forts of earth, and a great deal of fand, efpecially about the mountains called Jokells, which are continually covered with ice and fnow. Fiery eruptions from thefe mountains have fometimes occafioned great overflowings by melting the ice and fnow, which wafhed away all the mould upon the flopes of the mountains and the adjacent parts, leaving nothing but the bare fand. Afhes and calcined ftones are only found about Hecla, Krafle and fuch mountains as have burned with violence, and thrown up great quantities of bituminous matter. It cannot be faid that thefe mountains frequently emit fire ; no fuch thing having been perceived fince the year 1728. This happened at the Jokell Oraife, eaftward in the diftrict of Skaftefield, and two years before at Krafle in the north diftrict. Thofe that live near thefe mountains have learned by experience, that, when the ice and fnow fwell to fuch a pitch as to ftop up the holes from whence the fire iffues, the earth begins to fhake, and foon after fiery eruptions enfue. At the time of this writing, they were apprehenfive that the mountain in Skaftefield which burnt in the year 1728, would very foon difgorge flames again, having obferved that the ice and fnow covered the aperture, and confequently kept the air and vapours from having vent †.	The

* Mr. Anderfon fays this ifland appears like a calcined rock, being totally deftroyed by the many fiery eruptions from the mountains and the burning earth around them : for hardly any thing elfe is met with, but afhes of mountains, and no where fuch fand as in other places, being chiefly a compound of calcined ftones and afhes.
† The fame Author relates, that when the fnow melts, it flows from the mountains like a torrent, carrying with it huge pieces of ice, burnt matter and minerals, and

The fatal confequences of fuch eruptions cannot be beheld without the greateft horror. They are ufually attended with rapid torrents, pouring down from the mountains and wafhing away every thing before them. The people generally fave themfelves, and it very feldom happens that they do not efcape; as may appear from the mountain in Portlandfbay in the year 1721, which not lefs fuddenly than violently overflowed. This I fhall relate in its proper place; but not one perifhed. Two travellers who beheld this violent eruption retreated to the top of a higher mountain, where they were obliged to ftay a day and half. Afterwards they purfued their journey acrofs part of the mountain that had overflowed. No cattle were deftroyed by this accident. It is natural to fuppofe that wherever thefe overflowings reach, the earth muft be greatly damaged *: but thefe mountains are chiefly crouded in one tract of the ifland and the eruption ufually happens at the fame place.

An account of the overflowing of the Jokell Kotlegau, in 1721.

This happened in 1721, in the diftrict of Skaftefield to the fouth, at a mountain called Kotlegau, about 30 or 36 Englifh miles from the fea, near Portland's bay. After feveral warnings by fhocks of an earthquake, it firft difgorged fire which melted down the ice. A moft rapid torrent of water enfued †, bearing away with it an incredible quantity of fand and earth,

and overflowing and wafhing away every thing before it in a manner moft dreadful to behold, nothing being able, whether people, cattle or houfes to efcape, or withftand its fury.

* Mr. Anderfon obferves, that the united power of fire and water has totally deftroyed this country, and left it full of chafms and frightful rugged and torn mountains.

† The fame Author relates, that the violent force with which the air rufhed forth and expanded itfelf, tore away a great part of the mountain, and carried it not only fix miles to the fea-fide, but fix miles farther into the fea, and there left it ftanding: it was of fuch bulk that part of it was confiderably above the furface of the water. He likewife fays, that the afhes were fwept away by the wind, not only over the whole ifland, but many miles out at fea, and that all the fifh that lay a drying were totally fpoiled. The horfes and cattle had their mouths cut and feftered, and were otherwife much hurt the two following years by the afhes and fand that were fcattered about. He further adds, that the foot of the mountain took fire and fpread itfelf underground, taking a courfe of more than 100 miles, and continually burning for the fpace of a whole year. The Author of this Hiftory contradicts this account and affures us, that the mountain ftands 30 or 36 miles from the fea, that the rain wafhed all the duft and afhes away in one day, and that he never could find any one that could give any account of fubterraneous fires at that place.

I   and

and deſtroying all the ground it went over by waſhing away all
the mould. The intire current ruſhed with the ſame violence
into the ſea and filled it up like a hill, to near three miles diſtance
from the ſhore. It ſince gradually declined to its preſent condition, appearing not much above the ſurface of the water. Between this mountain and the ſea there is a rock called Haver Ey,
to the top of which the two travellers retired. Though the inundation overſpread all adjoining parts to the height of ſeveral fa-
thoms, and deſtroyed a deal of fine ground and graſs, they notwithſtanding, about a day and a half after, purſued their journey
acroſs the country that had been overflowed, and were able to
give the beſt account of this frightful ſight, which they beheld
without any danger from the top of the rock Haver Ey.

This mountain ſtands in an extenſive ſandy plain, called Mid-
dals Sand.

Many years before, the ſame misfortune happened to this
place and deſtroyed the valley, where there was good graſs.
The houſes that then ſtood thereon were intirely conſumed,
but it received no additional hurt this time, as being ruined before.
The prodigious quantity of ſand, ſtones, and earth, carried into
the ſea, may be aſcertained from what ſtill remains to be ſeen, as
alſo from the account given of the iſland of Weſtman, which
lies 72 miles out at ſea; where the ſea all of a ſudden roſe with
a violent motion to ſuch an uncommon height, that it was with
the greateſt difficulty, the fiſhermen ſaved their veſſels from
being toſſed aſhore, and waſhed over by the waves. Such a violent agitation of the ſea, and at ſuch a diſtance, ſufficiently proves
what an exceſſive quantity of ſand, &c. muſt have been poured
with the water into the ſea.

The fiery eruption, together with the aſhes, ſand, and ſmoke
that followed, ſo eclipſed the ſun, that it did not appear for a
whole day. The aſhes and ſand were carried to an incredible
diſtance, and almoſt to all parts of the iſland where the wind
blew. The graſs newly mowed, the hay that was out, and all
the fiſh that were hanging to dry, were covered by them: But
a day's rain waſhed all clean again. The fire only continued
flaming with this great violence at intervals. Whenever it ceaſed,
it was ſucceeded by thick dark ſmoke and vapour. Probably the

E

fire

fire was fmothered by the great quantity of melted fnow that poured in and occafioned this dark thick fteam. This inundation lafted about three days. It was dangerous travelling for a long while after. In many places fand covered the fnow and ice, and travellers funk through; but I do not find that any confiderable accident happened. In fuch a flood every thing mixed together, for when it fubfided all things were found promifcuoufly jumbled with one another.

An account of the eruption from the Jokell Oraife, in 1728.

As Jokell Kotlegau overflowed, fo did alfo, the Jokell, or mountain Oraife to the eaft of the diftrict of Skaftefield. The fire broke out between Ladyday and Midfummer, and continued burning till the beginning of October of the fame year. The water flowed from the mountain between two farmhoufes called Hoff and Sandfeld, which lie not above fix miles from the foot of the mountain, and about the fame diftance from each other. It fpread itfelf beyond thefe houfes in the flat country, and wafhed through the lower houfe and dairy, and carried off all the milk, butter, &c. the people faved themfelves by getting on the tops of the houfes. The water did not rife fo high, and only filled the infide. Numbers of the cattle from both farms were carried off, and fome of them were afterwards found parboiled. It ran along the vallies and emptied itfelf into the fea; but the ftones, fand and earth, carried away by the current were not any way equal in quantity, nor rufhed on fo violently as the former, though greater damages were fuftained. No cattle were loft in the other eruption, nor any field of grafs deftroyed, the fame being entirely demolifhed by former inundations: but the ftream of the eruption we are now talking of, paffed over fine fields, and deftroyed the better part of the cattle that were grazing in them.

This is a faithful relation of the whole hiftory of thefe two Jokells, which in 1721 and 1728, broke out in flames, and by melting vaft quantities of fnow and ice, occafioned very great inundations and all the dangerous confequences we have enumerated; by which providentially no human creature came to any hurt.

hurt. These mountains remain as they were, though the shocks of earthquakes and the heavy pieces of ice that fall and tear down from them heavy stones, may have altered their external form *. They must, no doubt, hereby receive great cracks and gaps, but it is certain they are not rent asunder.

Though the earth round these mountains seems not to be impregnated with sulphur, yet it is most likely that the interior parts of the mountains are full of such combustible matter, by reason of the violent fiery eruptions which happen. None of the adjoining mountains or the ground took fire, as at Krafle in the northern district. The ground there, it is well known, abounds with sulphur.

C H A P. VIII.

Concerning the mountain Hecla.

HECLA has always been famous for one of the most noted burning mountains in the known world. Some are of opinion that it has a communication with the mountain Vesuvius in Italy: for as soon as the one begins to disgorge flames, the other does the same.

At present, Hecla makes no great figure among the burning mountains in Iceland; having ceased to emit flames these many years: but others have exerted themselves as much as even Hecla has done, as Krafle in the northern district, and Kotlegau and Oraife in the district of Skaftefield. It likewise appears that Hecla has no kind of communication or connection with Ætna or Vesuvius: for these two mountains have lately burned and Hecla has been quiet. Certain it is, that Hecla has many times burned with great fury; but that it continued so for several hundred years together, is not to be credited. It cannot be said to burn continually, when many years have passed since it entirely ceased, and not the least symptom of fire or smoke appeared. During the term of the 800 years that Iceland has been inhabited, Hecla burned ten times, namely, in 1104, 1157, 1222, 1300, 1341, 1362, 1389, 1558, 1636, and 1693. This last time the flames appeared the 13th of February, and continued

---

* Mr. Anderson tells us this mountain stands 30 or 36 miles from the sea.

till

till the August following. In the same manner every other time, it continued burning several months together. By this account we see that in the 13th Century it was most disturbed, having broke out several times *. It afterwards ceased 169 years including the whole 14th century. In the 15th century, it burned but once, and in the 16th only twice. It now has been quiet upwards of 60 years; from whence I draw this inference, that by its gradual decrease the fire got vent in another place, broke out in some of the other mountains, and may probably entirely cease. Now not the least symptom of smoke or fire is perceptible. Some small cavities are discoverable in the rock, full of boiling hot water; but of this kind are many much more considerable in several parts of the island.

It is remarkable and worthy of observation; that the last time Hecla had an eruption, the country all around was strewed with sand, pumice-stone, and other bituminous matter. But length of time, rain and wind have gradually cleared the high ground and washed away this matter into low marshy places, which, by that means, have been dried up and now bear grass. The hills as if manured by it, are finer and fatter than ever, being now covered with the finest grass. In other places mould has gathered over the ashes a foot or two deep. At the foot of this mountain, there are houses and farms. Many people out of curiosity have gone to the top of this mountain. In the year 1750 two Icelanders, students in the university of Copenhagen, came home to make some physical observations. Arriving at this place they ascended the mountain, and found great heaps of ashes and sand, great cracks and chasms, and several cavities filled with boiling hot water. After they had tired themselves with walking in ashes and sand up to their knees, they came down safe and well, but very much fatigued. Many others have had the same curiosity, but none discovered the least appearance of fire or any thing burning. Hecla is a very high mountain, and one of the highest in the island. It is also what they call a Jockell; for the top, which none can come at, is continually covered with ice and snow.

* Mr. Anderson tells us it has burned successively for many hundred years, and that it is now only recovering itself to burn and disgorge with greater rage and fury.

The

The particulars of thefe eight chapters have been fet forth by other authors in fuch manner, as to convey to the readers ftrange ideas of this place, and very different from what I myfelf experienced. For the fatisfaction therefore of the public, I will in one chapter give a fuccinct and general defcription of this ifland and its properties, with regard to extent and the peculiar qualities of the earth, the mountains, and the foil, in order to place in a clearer light, and lay down more exact notions of what has already been but confufedly handled.

C H A P. IX.

*A brief and general defcription of Iceland with regard to its fize,
and the peculiar properties of the earth and mountains.*

ICELAND is one of the largeft iflands in Europe, and inferior in magnitude to none but the ifland of Great Britain. The length from eaft to weft I compute at about 720 Englifh miles, and the breadth upon an average about 300.

This great country is very uneven and has vaft ridges of mountains, both lengthways from eaft to weft, and acrofs the country. Between thefe mountains are fine and fruitful vallies, and fome very large openings feveral miles in length and breadth ; by which the country is divided into 18 fyffells or fhires, each of which is as extenfive as a province in Denmark, and fome are fo confiderable that two fyffelmænd, or juftices, are appointed for them. The fyffells or fhires are parted in feveral places by great lakes and rivers.

The mountains which lie in the midft of the ifland are exceeding rugged, barren and defolate ; though fome few among them are covered with grafs. The mountains that part the fhires, are for the better part very fruitful, and yield great plenty of excellent grafs. The barren mountains are of two kinds : the one, nothing but fand and ftone, the other vaft huge rocks, covered with ice and fnow all the year round, and diftinguifhed by the name Jokeler. Though continually covered with ice and fnow, they are not the higheft among the rocks. Some are rather low and furrounded by much loftier, on which the fnow melts away in the fummer. This muft be owing to fome pecu-

liar

liar quality in the nature of the foil. From thofe barren defolate mountains fire will fometimes break forth, and chiefly from thofe called Jokells, such as Hecla, Kotlegau and Oraife. As for Krafle in the northern diftrict, it never was a Jokell or perpetually covered with ice and fnow.

Along the country are feveral ridges of rocks, between which are large vallies, but not fo deep as thofe towards the fea fide, being rather upon a level with the mountains that lie nearer the fea. However, thefe vallies are deep in proportion to the high mountains that furround them, as may appear by travelling into the heart of the country, the afcent being continual and, as it were, infenfible. The heart of the country is entirely uninhabited, though containing many very fine and fruitful fpots, where fheep are often kept to feed all the year round, and fometimes feveral years together; expofed to all forts of weather without ever being houfed. When thefe fheep are driven away to be fent to market, they are found exceeding fine and fat, and by far better than thofe kept about the farms in other vallies. Here are alfo pleafant rivulets, brooks and ponds of fine clear and good water, and quantities of fine fifh. The large vallies which are inhabited, lie all much lower than thofe up the country, gradually defcending to the fea fide. Some extend along the coaft, and may be about 25 or 30 miles in breadth towards the mountains. Others again run in between the mountains. All of the feveral tracts that conftitute properly the fhires, have fmall vallies between the hills for the grazing of cattle, and in the fummer-feafon huts are built, where proper perfons are appointed to manage and look after the milk, butter, wool, &c.

From fome of the mountains flow large and fmall rivers, befides rivulets and ftreams, all which water the flat or low country, and abound with very fine fifh. There are alfo many bays, creeks and harbours towards the fea, very convenient for fifhing, and up the country fine large lakes 30 or 36 miles in circumference, and fome lefs, which abound with moft excellent fifh. Thus the inhabitants are not in want of many good conveniencies for nourifhment and fubfiftence. Woods are fcarce, though there are fome few, chiefly in the northern diftrict, but in no proportion to thofe other countries are productive of. As to the foil,

it

it differs as in most countries. Fine mould is found in some places, clayey and sandy ground in some others, besides very large bogs, or marshes commonly overflowed with water, though in the summer they dry up and may be rode over. These marshes, when drained, become very fine grounds. Turf is found almost every where, and in some places exceeding good.

The disadvantages that attend this country are chiefly the following. Burning mountains, which occasioned conflagrations of the earth, as already related in discoursing of the mountain of Krafle, where the earth abounds with sulphur. When the Jokells take fire, they occasion great inundations, by melting the vast quantity of ice. and snow with which they are covered, as has been seen in the account of Skaftefield. These two calamities, God be praised, happen but seldom, and cause not such havock as represented by some authors and travellers. As an account of the excellencies of this country, its fine fisheries, its breeding of cattle and many other things of note, require more room than is intended in this short and general description, I shall treat more at large of the same in their proper places. However, I thought it not improper to give a short sketch of the face of the country, the mountains, rocks, valleys, &c. so much the more, as some authors and travellers have most unmercifully pictured their description like hell itself, and consequently transmitted to the public a very false and wretched idea of the country. I shall therefore now proceed according to my first intention, which was to discuss and elucidate each subject in a separate article.

CHAP. X.

Concerning a lake which takes fire three times a year.

ABOUT Hecla are several little springs, and at the foot of the mountain several ponds, both perpetually hot, and some hotter than others. I do not find that any one with a thermometer has made experiments whether they are hotter in winter than summer; or whether they are of an equal heat all the year round. Certain it is, that sometimes a stronger steam arises from them than at other times. This I have observed my self; and it is known by experience, that when the steam or

vapour

vapour is very thick it is likely to be rainy and damp weather, and vice versâ, when the air is fine and clear, it is by far less dense, and the steam does not rise so fast. But neither here, nor at any —other of the hot springs, of which there are many, have ever any flames been seen *. The smoke or steam, as before observed, is sometimes stronger but not periodical. Two opposite elements will not unite in this country no more than in any other. Those that made this relation happened to come a day too late and only found the water smoking, which may be seen in many hundred parts of the island, as also some very strange and surprizing phænomena, which I shall treat of in the next article.

C H A P. XI.

Concerning the hot waters.

HOT waters are found in many parts of this island. But though a physical disquisition be not the plan I lay down for myself, yet I presume the same causes assigned by philosophers in other countries may be allowed here. I have visited many of these warm baths, but never found the least appearance of sulphur in the ground near them ; nor do the waters taste of any mineral, which I tried by several experiments. Where these hot springs are, there is frequently a small bason at the place they flow out, which may contain about twenty or thirty gallons. In some places the water that runs from the rocks over hot grounds is heated to such a degree as to send forth smoke or steam: but these can hardly be called brooks. The ground does not smoke, though so hot, that it would be impossible to stand upon it without shoes. This I have observed in a dry summer when the waters above were dried up. Where I found these hot grounds, it has been chiefly stony, with small cracks about the breadth of the little finger. From thence the heat has been much stronger than from other places. When the

---

* Mr. Anderson tells us that about three English miles from Hecla there is a small fresh-water lake always warm, rather hotter in the winter, and according to the accounts of the people in the neighbourhood, endowed with the peculiar property of taking fire three times a year, and burning about a fortnight together in small bright flames. When they go out, it steams or smokes for several days after. He adds, that his factor went on purpose to see this strange phænomenon, but that it happened to go out the day before he arrived.

water runs over these narrow cracks it boils up stronger than elsewhere. These hot waters are called in the native language Hver, and in Iceland confist of three sorts. Some moderately hot that a person may hold his hand in; others boiling hot, and others that boil to such a degree, as to throw the water up like a fountain. Of the last are two sorts, some that boil promiscuously throwing up the water in a common manner; others that clear at certain intervals and afterwards in a regular order throw up the water. Of the latter sort that in the district of Huusevig, is the most remarkable in the country; a short description of it, will not, I presume, be disagreeable.

CHAP. XII.

A short description of a hot spring in the district of Huusevig.

THIS extraordinary spring is to be met with in the north shire and parish of Huusevig near a farm called * Reykum, about 50 or 60 miles from the mountain Krafle, which has been before spoken of. At this place are three springs which lie about 30 fathom from each other. The water boils up in them by turns in the following manner. When the spring or well at one end has thrown up its water, then the middle one begins, which subsiding, that at the other end rises, and after it the first begins again, and so on in the same order by a continued succession, each boiling up three times in about a quarter of an hour. They are all in a flat open place, but the ground hard and rocky. In two of them the water rises between the cracks and boils up about two feet only above the ground. The third has a large round aperture, by which it empties itself into a place like a bason, as if formed by art, in a hard stone rock, and as big as a brewing copper. On discharging itself here, it will rise at the third boiling ten or twelve feet high above the brim, and afterwards sink four feet or more in the bason or reservoir. At this interval it may be approached near enough, to see how deep it sinks; but those that have this curiosity, must take care to get away before it

* By such like names many are called in this island, because they adopt the name of the springs they lie near: for Reyk in the Iceland language signifying smoke, the farm is therefore so called from the smoke and steams that arise out of these springs.

boils

boils up again. As foon as it has funk to the deepeft ebb, it immediately rifes again, and that in three boilings. At the firft, it rifes half way up to the edge or brim; in the fecond, above the brim; in the third, as before obferved, 10 or 12 feet high. Then it finks at once four feet below the brim of the refervoir, and when funk here, rifes at the other end, and from thence proceeds to the middle one, and fo on by a conftant regular rotation.

Having now given a defcription of thefe fprings and the furprizing manner of their rifing, I fhall add a fhort account of fome extraordinary effects of the water. If the water out of the largeft well is poured into bottles it will ftill continue to boil up twice, or thrice, and at the fame time with the water in the well. Thus long will the effervefcence continue after the water is taken out of the well, but this being over it foon quite fubfides and grows cold. If the bottles are corked up the moment they are filled, fo foon as the water rifes in the well they burft in pieces: this experiment has been proved on many fcore bottles, to try the effects of the water. Whatever is caft into the well when the water fubfides, it attracts with it down to the bottom, even wood, which on another like fluid would float: but when the water flows again, it throws every thing up, which may be found at the fide of the bafon. This has been often tried with ftones as large and as heavy as the ftouteft fellows have hardly been able to tumble in. Thefe ftones made a violent noife on being plunged to the bottom; but when the water rofe again, they were ejaculated with force beyond the edge of the well. A vaft many ftones lie about that have been ufed in fuch experiments. The water by continually flowing over, has formed a little brook, which, it feems, grows cool by degrees, and at laft falls into a little river. It is a pleafant water to drink, when cold, and hardly taftes of any mineral. On the neighbouring plain there is generally a very fine growth of grafs, but within three or four yards of thefe wells, or fprings, the place being continually wet by the fplafhing of the water, all the mould is wafhed away, and nothing but the naked ftone rock appears. There is a farm at a fmall diftance and clofe by it this water runs from the well. It is is here but juft warm. The cattle water in it, and the cows yield a much greater quantity of milk than others that do not

5

water

water at that place. This is a thing univerfally known, and is a very extraordinary effect of the water. Such are the ftrange and remarkable properties of thefe wells or fprings, of which there are feveral others much of the fame kind, but the alternate boiling up of the water is intirely peculiar to thefe three. Where any of thefe hot fprings are, they continually exhale a vapour or fteam, which is greater or lefs according as the water is agitated, or the air lighter or heavier. This fteam is fometimes feen at a very great diftance.

The ufe the inhabitants make of thefe fprings.

They that live near thefe hot baths, of which in this ifland there are many, whofe water is continually boiling hot, employ the fame for feveral ufes. They fometimes take a pot or any veffel filled with cold water, put the meat or whatever they have to boil in it, and hang the veffel at a certain depth in the well *. It prefently boils, and in this manner they drefs their boiled victuals without being at any expence for fuel.

I have met with travellers, who having their tea-kettle with them, filled it with water and boiled it inftantly in one of thefe. baths; and I have feen people fit the whole day bending of hoops for barrels at the edge of thefe boiling hot baths, by the heat of which they bent fome of an extraordinary thicknefs. Every two hours or lefs, they were obliged to fet afide their work, and take frefh air to prevent any ill effects from the fulphureous and other bad fmells of the fteam, which expands itfelf to a confiderable diftance. The ftench has been fo ftrong at fome of them, that I was not able to bear it. The ground about thefe hot wells is generally of various colours, and contains fome fulphur, alum and faltpetre.

Befides the benefit the inhabitants have of boiling their victuals and water at thefe places, they make ufe of them to wafh or bathe in. The water that continually overflows and runs at fome diftance is of proper heat for bathing. Sometimes they contrive to bring cold water to the bafons : for as before obferved, there are actually bafons at the mouth of fome of the fprings, as if they were hewn out and fafhioned by a ftone-cutter. By this means they affuage the heat of the water, and make it fit for

* Mr. Anderfon tells us they faften their meat to a piece of wood and dip it in the hot well till it is boiled.

bathing.

bathing. I have feen one of thefe bafons moft remarkably capa-
cious, fmooth within, and well fhaped for the purpofe. It was
in a folid rock without any cracks, the bottom very fmooth, and
at any time could be covered with a tilt-cloth. It had befides
this advantage; that there was an aqueduct to it from hot and
cold fprings, fome fo hot that one could not bear a finger in
them, others fo cold as ice, and both conveyed to or from the
bafon at pleafure, by which means the water in the bafon could
be brought to any defired degree of warmth. At the bottom of
this refervoir, fo formed by nature, was a hole made, through
which the water could eafily be carried off into a little adjoining
rivulet. A frefh fupply of clean water was always at hand to
fill it again on ftopping up the hole. The people that live here,
bathe frequently in it, and chiefly on this account are a very
healthy people, and generally live to a good old age.

The common people are full of a fuperftitious notion that
fome ftrange birds are continually hovering and harbouring about
thefe hot wells †.

They relate this, as matter of fact, and believe it, though on
hear-fay only from their fathers and great-grand fathers; but
upon enquiry not one is to be met with, that ever faw any of
thefe ftrange birds.

Befides, it is highly improbable, that birds fhould harbour
about or fwim on water, fo hot, that a piece of beef may be
boiled in it. Very likely birds may refort to the water that overflows and runs in a continued ftream, cooling by degrees, and
at laft emptying itfelf into fome river: but it cannot be faid that
birds particularly harbour about any of thefe places. In the rivers,
which the different ftreams of thefe hot wells flow into, is found
the fame kind of fifh, as in moft other rivers; fuch as, falmon,
trout and a variety of other fifh, which is a convincing proof
that the waters have no ftrong mineral quality in them, it being
known by experience, that fifh will not live in water that is any
way tinctured with fulphur, or any other mineral quality.

The waters in general are very good in this ifland; but this
is not owing to any mineral quality in them, having found my-

---

† Mr. Anderfon fays there is a fort of black-birds with long bills, much like a
fnipe, continually harbouring about thefe hot wells.

self

felf by repeated experiments, that they retain but very little of any mineral, except in a few parts; where they feem impregnated with fmall portions of a chalybeat, or vitriolic fubftance *. In moft places they are quite pure, without the leaft foreign tincture any way difcoverable by common experiments, or by the tafte. It is therefore evident, that the earth all over the ifland does not abound with fulphur, faltpetre, and other falts; the waters in the diftrict, as I have before related, where the ground is full of fulphur, have a ftrong fulphureous tafte and fmell †.

CHAP. XII.

Concerning the property and quality of the rocks and mountains, in which probably marble may be found.

WHAT has been already faid concerning the rocks and mountains in Iceland, might feem more than fufficient, had not my defign been to enter into a proper detail of things. However, to avoid unneceffary repetitions, I refer my readers to what has been faid before on this fubject, wherein I prefume, I made it appear, that many of thefe mountains yield great ftore of very good grafs. As to their containing marble, I will not pretend that I ever difcovered any. 'Tis true, that along the coaft I found ftones of very beautiful colours, fome red, fome greenifh, and others finely variegated: the fame I alfo found in fome of the mountains; but none of them are marble ftones, though it is very probable, that marble may be found in the ifland ‡. His Danifh majefty fent miners there to break the rocks and make experiments. The natives, will, no doubt, reap fome advantage from their inftructions, and in procefs of time, probably marble, and other valuable minerals may be difcovered.

* Mr. Anderfon fays that moft of the fprings in this ifland both hot and cold, are good and wholfome waters, becaufe all, more or lefs, contain fome mineral quality.
† The fame Author here again alledges, that the whole country abounds with fulphur, and that a fpade cannot be put half way into the ground, but it brings up fulphur inftead of mould.
‡ This Author fays on this head, that the mountains and hills are nothing but fand and ftones, tho' he allows, that, in all probability, marble may be found in the rocks, becaufe found both in Sweden and Norway. He adds, that fome ftones found along the coaft may be deemed a fpecies of marble.

C H A P. . XIII.

Concerning cryſtals.

CRYSTALS are ſometimes found here, but as they never happened to fall in my way, I will not take upon me to aſſert or deny that there is any ſuch thing *. The peculiar property of·that which goes under the denomination of Chryſtallus Iſlandica, conſiſts in repreſenting the object, ſeen through it, double. But this is not properly what is commonly called cryſtal, though it retains that appellation. It is nothing but ſpar, and is ſaid to be found eaſtward, on a mountain near Rodefiord. Very likely it may ; but as I have not been eaſtward, I cannot vouch for the truth of this aſſertion.

C H A P. XIV.

Concerning pumice ſtone.

WHERE vulcano's or burning mountains are, there pumice ſtone is generally found. Whether that which is found here is clean or foul I cannot determine, being unacquainted with the properties it ſhould have to be deemed good and clean †.

C H A P. XV.

Concerning the metallic ores found in this country.

THERE are not only grounds to preſume that there are ores and minerals in the Iceland mountains, but very ſufficient demonſtration ; it being very well known, that the country people frequently find great lumps of ore, ſo rich, that a common wood fire will melt them. Of this ore they themſelves have caſt ſeals and buttons, ſome of which have been found to

---

* Mr. Anderſon ſays that the cryſtal found in Iceland is very ſoft, friable, and unfit for any manufacture.
† The ſame Author tells us, that two ſorts of pumice ſtone are here found, the one grey, the other black. Both, in his opinion, are foul. This ſtone is diſgorged in the eruption of burning mountains.

be

be pure filver. Many of the inhabitants for foldering the ward of a key, will go into the field to feek after a kind of ftuff, which they know will anfwer the purpofe. Having applied it to the place they want to have faftened, they put clay round it, and throw it into the fire till they think it has received fufficient heat. Then they take it out, ftrike off the clay, and find the parts ftrongly foldered together. What can this be they find in the field, unlefs pieces of ore that contain a metal proper to folder with ? Probably it is copper-ore, that metal being fit for foldering iron. It is certainly known, that many places are remarkable for being productive of very rich copper-ore. Several of the inhabitants have prepared for themfelves various utenfils of iron, made out of an ore which they find in abundance, without any great trouble, in many places. Hence it is plain, that the ifland contains not only iron, but other valuable metals *. Probably a time may come when fome will undertake to fearch for thefe hidden treafures. Nothing is likely to obftruct the enterprize but the fcarcity of wood; but if the mines fhould be found rich enough to defray the expences, this obftruction may be eafily removed. Great things, in my opinion, may therefore be expected from the Iceland ore, and fo much the more, as pure metal of the aforefaid three forts, has often been found above ground †.

C H A P. XVI.

Concerning rofin and turf.

IT is not to be queftioned, but that the Iceland mountains contain rofin, pitch, and other bituminous matter. This is demonftrable by the mountains, which fometimes have taken fire, as it muft be fomething of this kind that feeds the fire fo long, efpecially where it takes a courfe over the ground for feveral miles. Turf is in plenty, and in the fouthern parts, the beft I

---

* Mr. Anderfon intimates, that there is no judging what metals may be found, none having ever given themfelves the trouble to look after any fuch thing.
† The fame Author affigns two reafons, the firft, that the mountains are frightful and dangerous; the fecond, that there is too great a fcarcity of timber for erecting works, and going through the operations of fmelting, refining, &c.

have

have ever feen *. The inhabitants in thofe parts where it is to be found, hardly burn any thing elfe. In other places they burn brufh-wood and furze, of which there is great plenty almoft every where. They cut alfo a fort of turf at low water along the fhore. It is black and heavy, and much the fame as the other on land. In the fouth parts they ufe much of this, either to fave the grafs turf, which is fcarcer there than in other places, or to fave themfelves the trouble of going far to fetch it, which thofe that live along the coaft would otherwife be neceffitated to do.

C H A P. XVII.

Concerning agates.

ICELAND produces two forts of agate. The one will burn like a candle, and is in fact a fpecies of bitumen. The other, which the Icelanders call Hrafn tinna (black flint ftone) does not burn. It is harder than the former, and will break in-to thin flakes, which are very tranfparent, and not unlike glafs. This makes me think it is a vitrification, and as great quantities of it is found about Krafle in the northern diftrict, it confirms me the more in my opinion. At this place pieces are found as large as a fmall fized table, and fome have weighed 100 or 120 pounds and upwards. The natives fet apart the firft fort, or inflamma-ble agate for fome fuperftitious ceremonies, which are conducted in the fame manner, as is defcribed in Cæfius *de mineralibus.* Others reject this ufe, and abhor all fuch practices.

C H A P. XVIII.

Concerning fulphur.

PURE native fulphur is not to be found any where above ground, fo as to be fcraped up and gathered. The earth being neither good nor fruitful where it is; the chief fign for difcovering it, is a ftrong heat underneath that fmokes through the

---

* Mr. Anderfon fays there is not much turf in this country, and in the fouth-ern parts very indifferent, becaufe it is full of fulphur, ftinks abominably, and waftes away too faft; but again he contradicts himfelf, for he fays at Hafnefiord it is very good, being black, heavy and firm.

ground.

ground. Generally speaking, where the foil is of this kind, there alſo are hot ſprings. Sulphur is equally found in the rocks, mountains and plains. Sometimes it ſhoots to a very conſiderable diſtance from the foot of the mountains *. There is always a lay of barren earth upon the ſulphur, which is properly nothing but ſand and clay. This ſame earth is of ſeveral colours, white, yellow, green, red and blue. When this lay is removed the ſulphur lies underneath, and may be taken up with ſhovels. By frequently digging as deep as a man's middle, the ſulphur is found in proper order. They ſeldom dig deeper, becauſe the place is generally too hot, and requires too much labour, as alſo, becauſe ſulphur may be had at an eaſier rate, and in greater plenty, in the proper places. Fourſcore horſes may be loaded in an hour's time, each horſe carrying 250 pounds weight. The beſt veins of ſulphur are known by a kind of bank or riſing in the ground, which is cracked in the middle. From hence a thicker vapour iſſues, and a greater heat is felt than in any other part. Theſe are the places they chooſe for digging, and after removing a layer or two of earth they come to the ſulphur, and find it beſt juſt under the bank or riſing of the ground, where it looks like candid ſugar. The farther from the middle of the bank the more it crumbles, at laſt appearing like mere duſt, which may be ſhovelled up. But the middle of the bank is an intire hard lump, and with difficulty broken through. The looſe duſt is likewiſe good ſulphur, but not quite ſo good as the hard lumps. In this manner they follow the vein, and when exhauſted, look out for another, of which there are plenty in that part of the country, as I before obſerved. The labourers not being able to bear this work in hot weather, chooſe the nights, which are light enough here in the midſt of ſummer to do any labour in. When they dig, they are obliged to tye woollen rags about their ſhoes to keep them from burning. The brimſtone when firſt taken out, is ſo hot that it can hardly be handled, but

* Mr. Anderſon tells us, that native ſulphur grows every where under the upper lay of mould, eſpecially in fenny and marſhy grounds. Frequently whole lumps are found as big as a man's fiſt, and it breaks out of the rocks ſo thick, that every two or three years it may be ſcraped off with irons and gathered; but our author aſſures us, that ſulphur entirely deſtroys the fertility of the earth, and that it is quite inconſiſtent that ſulphur, which requires hot and dry grounds, ſhould ever be produced in bogs and marſhes.

grows

grows cooler by degrees. In two or three years thefe veins are filled with fulphur again, the mines being always quick with a furprizing vegetation. This is the genuine nature and difpofition of the fulphur in this ifland, with all the circumftances relating to the digging and gathering of it *. From the year 1722, to the year 1728, fulphur was taken out of the veins, and exported to foreign parts, with the confent, and to the great advantage of the inhabitants ; but a fhip having fince been caft away near the harbour, the cargo, which was fulphur, fo affected the water for a confiderable time, that no fifh were feen in it. The inhabitants being ftill defirous of turning this commodity to fome account, continued gathering and tranfporting it to the trading towns, till fuch time as the merchants would not take any more from them. Thus it was, that thofe who had a third fhare in this concern, and had ordered large quantities to be gathered, loft very confiderably by it, being never able to difpofe of it. A great many more of the inhabitants fuffered in the fame manner ; for when they had often gathered it, by not being able to difpofe of it at market, vaft quantities were wafted. In reality, it was not owing to the inhabitants that this fulphur trade ceafed, a thing very much to be pitied ; but, I prefume, I can in fome meafure affign the caufe, which was the death of the perfon at Copenhagen, who had the fole and exclufive privilege. This death happening foon after he obtained the fame, put a ftop to the concern, and no one fince has taken it up, perhaps for want of knowledge and experience to fet it on a proper footing. That fifh have an averfion to fulphur is not at all ftrange, there being feveral inftances to confirm this opinion, among which may be alledged, the fhip at Huufevig that was caft away with its cargo of fulphur; the matter that flowed into the lake of My-vatne from the burning mountain called Krafle, and the boat that was employed in putting the fulphur on board the fhip in Huufevig's harbour, which could never afterwards be ufed for fifhing.

* Mr. Anderfon tells us, that they now leave off gathering fulphur, as they did feveral times before, having found it very hurtful to their fifheries, which are their principal fupport.

CHAP.

CHAP. XIX.

Concerning falt, whether any be found in Iceland.

IT is more than I can pretend to fay, that common falt is not to be found in Iceland. Whoever pofitively afferts that it is not, muft have traverfed the whole country, and be poffef-fed of the knowledge and experience requifite to examine into the matter, and to make the neceffary experiments for a convincing proof*. It is true, that having no where myfelf met with falt-fprings, or rock-falt, (fal petræ) I can only fay, that upon a fpecimen of the latter being fhewed me, I was affured, that there are great quantities in a certain part of the ifland, which is very probable. That there are falt fprings about this ifland at fome diftance in the fea is pretty certain, and it is very probable, that fuch are in the country. I have obferved in feveral places along the coaft, after a high flood, and the water being cleared off again, that the moifture, when dried up by the fun, left a cruft of falt all about the rocks, which the people being very watchful of, fcrape off, and gather for the ufe of their families. Thus it cannot pofitively be faid, that no common falt is found in the ifland. Moreover it may appear from ancient grants to the church in the catholic times, that falt works and other privileges, particularly northward, were affigned for foul-maffes to certain ecclefiaftics and monafteries; by which it is demonftrable, that in former times they made falt; for the ec-clefiaftics not eafily fatisfied with titular gifts and privileges, muft have the fubftance and not the fhadow. Two gentle-men having here made experiments on fea-water, I was affured by one of them, that one tun of French falt which he boiled in fea water, produced one tun and a quarter of good white falt. This was done without the proper boilers and other vehi-cles for this purpofe, and without any other knowledge of the matter than what common reafon dictated. By this alone we may fee, that it is not impoffible to make falt in Iceland.

* Mr. Anderfon fays, there is no common falt to be found in any part of this ifland.

CHAP.

CHAP. XX.

Concerning forests and trees.

I BEFORE obſerved, that foreſts and wood are ſcarce in this country, yet not ſo very ſcarce as ſome travellers have repreſented. In the north diſtrict is a wood called Fnioſkadal, about four Engliſh miles and a half long. In the ſame diſtrict are ſeveral of the kind; and but few farms there, are without a little adjoining nurſery of young trees, ſome as thick as an arm *. This north diſtrict, which is alſo called to this day the diſtrict of Thingöe, from an iſland ſo called, where formerly aſſizes uſed to be held, has, beſides the aforeſaid Fnioſkadal, another pretty large wood, by name Aaſkov, and ſeveral others leſs conſiderable †. There is a wood as large as either of the former eaſtward, in the diſtrict of Mule, which is called Hallormſtade, and another in the ſouth quarter in the diſtrict of Borgefiord, called Huuſefell ‡. It is therefore plain, that there are many woods in the ſeveral quarters and diviſions of this iſland; but in proportion to its extent and bigneſs, it may with a deal of juſtneſs be ſaid, that there is a ſcarcity. However, this want is compenſated in ſeveral places, by the great quantities of fine large timber, that every year comes floating aſhore. Of this they have more than they know what to do with; for being under no neceſſity to conſume it, they let it lie in heaps and rot, not having veſſels to tranſport it to their fellow-countrymen, who want it in other parts of the iſland. Beſides the woods already mentioned, ſhrubs and buſhes lie ſcattered about, ſome high enough to ſhade one from the ſun. Theſe ſhrubs conſiſt for the better part of juniper and blackberry buſhes, of which the people burn charcoal for their

---

* Mr. Anderſon ſays, that there are no trees in the whole iſland, except in the northern part; but that a Copenhagen merchant told him, that between Huuſvig and Olfiord (rather Oefiord) about 36 Engliſh miles diſtant from each other, he came into a wood four or five Engliſh miles long.

† The ſame Author ſays he was informed, that near Thingöre abbey, there is a ſmall wood chiefly of birch trees; but he confounds Thingöre abbey with Thingöe.

‡ He alſo alledges, that in other parts of the iſland, there are only to be ſeen along the rivers a few low water willows, and blackberry and juniper-berry buſhes, of which the inhabitants are very ſaving, uſing them only to burn charcoal of for their forges.

forges.

forges. The numerous families in this island, and all those that live near the sea coast, have boats, houses, chests, cupboards, &c. with doors, locks and keys, and as I before observed, live at such distance from each other, that they cannot easily lend a mutual assistance; for which reason they are obliged to keep in their houses an apparatus for various sorts of mechanical functions, and though ever so poor, have at least a smith's forge, which they cannot dispense with *. The smith's work they do themselves, every one as well as he can, as also every other kind of mechanical business, they are under a necessity of performing. There is some reason to think, that in ancient days there was no scarcity of wood in this island. This I cannot ascertain for fact; because not the least sign appears that ever pine or fir-trees grew in this island, though the forests in the northern and much colder countries generally consist of pine and fir-trees. No other kind of trees but birch is seen; perhaps the seed of the former was never brought here; for I presume that there is no room to doubt, but that they would have grown here as well as in more severe climates. In several places, roots of trees have been found in the ground; from whence it may be supposed with good reason, that in former days woods stood in the parts that are now plains, without a tree to be seen †. A very extraordinary sort of wood, which they call forte brand, or black brand, very hard, heavy and black, like ebony, is found somewhat deep in the ground, in broad, thin, and pretty long pannels or leaves, fit for a moderate size table. It is generally wavy or undulated, and is always found between the rocks or great stones, wedged, as it were, quite close in. At first, on considering its situation, I was very doubtful whether it was wood or a petrification; but as it could be planed and managed in every respect like wood, the shavings also having the appearance of such, I was induced to think that it is nothing but wood. However, as a very extraordinary phænomenon, it may deserve a longer dissertation than this historical account will admit of.

* Mr. Anderson says there are but very few smiths forges in the island.
† The same Author says, a kind of very hard rotten wood is found under ground.

CHAP.

CHAP. XXI.

Concerning the pasture-land and grass.

ALL over the island are seen spacious tracts, that yield plenty of fine grass for feeding of cattle, which are here kept during the whole summer, till the severe cold weather comes in [*]. In some places, though left out all the year round, and for years together, they grow exceeding fat, and as fine as can be wished. The reason why the several districts of the north country have the greatest reputation for breeding of cattle, is, because the inhabitants make it their chief trade; those of other parts of the island relying more on their fisheries, and some entirely depending upon fishing, whereby they neglect the breeding of cattle, though they have as fine grass, and as good conveniencies for this purpose as any in the north. Rather than to attribute this to neglect, properly speaking, the inhabitants are too few to attend both articles. It is certain, that the grass grows faster in the north country than in the south; for sometimes the snow hardly disappearing till midsummer, no grass is observed to sprout up; but in about 12 or 14 days after, it grows near two foot high, exceeding fine, and fit to be mowed. This probably may be accounted for from the snow's continually covering the ground, and warming, and defending it from the frost. In the midst of summer also, the sun (in this latitude) continues so long above the horizon, that vegetation is thereby greatly promoted. The same cannot be said of the south parts, where the snow not constantly covering the earth, they must naturally be liable to the usual injuries of frosts. Besides what has been related of the manner they keep their cattle, by sending them to pasture in the mountains, at some distance from their farms and habitations, it is to be understood, that none are kept at home, or near their houses, which they generally contrive to build on or near a fertile spot of ground, somewhat remote from the

---

[*] Mr. Anderson says, that though the lay of mould that covers the rocks, sand, sulphur, stones, &c. be very thin, yet very good pasture-land is met with, especially in the northern countries along the rivers and lakes, the grass growing there a foot high.

mountains,

mountains. Every farm has such a field or piece of ground, which the Icelanders calls Tun. It is watched by dogs, that none of the cattle may come near it. They manure it in the best manner they respectively can afford for the producing of grafs, which they mow down, and reserve for a winter supply. As for the grafs that grows in the mountains, they always let the cattle eat it, and never cut any down *. These (Tuner) or meadows, are generally very clear from rocks or stones. Many, no doubt, of them (for they cannot be all alike) are uneven and have a great many little hillocks and stones upon them, together with rocks rising out of the ground; but it cannot be said, that all are indiscriminately so, or that the country is all over craggy and rugged; for even in the very mountains are found large and fine fertile plains, which are never mowed, though not any wise incumbered with stones or hillocks. They cut down their grafs, and get in their hay with as much ease as any where in Denmark. They also use the same instruments. Their scythes 'tis true, are not quite so long, neither is the blade so broad, by reason of their not having it in their power to manage such long ones in hilly or stony grounds. With those they use, they dispatch a great deal of work, one man being able to cut down 30 square fathom a day.

CHAP. XXII.

Whether there are wholsome herbs and roots in this island.

AMONG the several herbs and roots of the growth of this island, and very beneficial to the health of the human body, is the *Cochlearia* and *Acetosa*, with many others. A botanist would certainly find here very good amusement. I must not omit mentioning the angelica root, which is found in abundance, and of an uncommon size and goodness. Some places produce such great quantities of it, that the inhabitants use it for food, and it agrees extremely well with them. They have no no-

---

* Mr. Anderson says, that what the cattle and sheep leave in the fields, is cut and gathered for the winter, but in a painful and toilsome manner, the ground being so uneven, full of mole-hills, stones and rubbish, that they cannot make use of a scythe to cut it down, but must use a small hand sickle, with which they carefully cut the grafs between the hillocks, stones, and little rocks.

tion

tion of taking any of thefe things by way of medicine, being a very healthy people, and as little afflicted with difeafes as
any nation whatever *. They make no great ufe of cochlearia,
but of acetofa they do, to mix with their drink, which is the
whey of four milk, and called by them Syre. This herb or root
they put to it merely to increafe the quantity. It is an adulteration, as they call it; for when this herb is mixed with the
whey, it will not keep; for which reafon, they fay their good
whey is adulterated by it. Thus they make no great account of
ufing it, neither do they think it wholfome, but rather a deceit,
or only out of neceffity. There is another herb called *Mufcus
Catharcticus Iflandiæ*, or mountain grafs, which they cook up
into a delicate difh. I have often eat of it; at firft out of curiofity, but afterwards for its palateablenefs and wholfomnefs †.
The excellent qualities of this herb are defcribed in the memoirs
of the fociety of arts and fciences in Sweden. It grows in great
abundance, and thofe that live near the places where it grows,
gather great quantities for their own ufe, and to fend to market.
People that live at a great diftance will fend and fetch horfe loads
away. Many ufe no meal or flower at all, when they are ftocked with this herb, which in every refpect is good and wholfome
food. It is a fort of mofs, and only grows on the rocks. There
is another herb confounded with this, called Fiöru-grafs. It is
a fea weed, thrown up by the fea, and found at low water.
The cattle are fond of it, and it is gathered by the inhabitants
at ebb tide, which Icelanders call Fiöre, from whence this weed
has the name of Fiöre-grafs.

C H A P. XXIII.

Concerning the fruits of the earth.

A L L kinds of things may be produced fit for a kitchen-
garden, and brought to proper maturity, and why not;
for this ifland is as proper for vegetation as Norway, having large

* Mr. Anderfon fays, that God's providence caufes a great quantity of wholfome
and medicinal herbs to grow here, fuitable to the climate, and the difeafes of the
country.

† The fame Author fays he has been told of an herb found only in a few places,
of which his author could neither give him the name, nor defcription, further than
that when boiled in milk, it taftes like a millet pudding.

plains

plains and fields, and a great deal of good ground *. With regard to the climate and piercing north winds, I will refer my
readers to the meteorological obfervations I made there two years
fucceffively. Thefe obfervations may be feen in the conclufion
of this work. By them, I am fatisfied, it will plainly appear,
that the cold during thefe two winters, in the fouth part of the
country, was not feverer than at Copenhagen. Nay, I queftion
if the weather is not often colder there. How far thofe piercing north winds extend, may likewife be feen in the tables of
thefe meteorological obfervations. The laft winter I made thefe
obfervations in, was reckoned by the inhabitants much feverer
than the winters in general are. It is plain, from what I have
related, that there is nothing here to obftruct vegetation, more
than in Norway or Denmark. In the year 1749, when I
came to Beffefted, one of his majefty's palaces or feats in Iceland, I found the garden in excellent order, and full of all kinds
of vegetables fit for a kitchen, fuch as parfley, fallary, thyme,
marjoram, cabbage, parfnips, carrots, turnips, peas, beans, in
fhort, all forts of greens wanted in a family. I can vouch with
the greateft truth, that I never faw a garden with better things
of the kind in it. They were all of good growth, and had all
the properties that good garden ftuff ought to have. They were
alfo in fuch plenty, that confiderable parcels of them were dried,
and laid by for the winter, fuch as fugar-peas, and the like. I
myfelf have taken up a turnip that weighed two pounds and a half.
Hereby I do not intimate that all were fo big, but only that they
are of a very good fize. They have goofeberry bufhes that produce fine and ripe berries. Thus there is no manner of doubt,
but that various fruit trees would bear here, and bring their fruit
to maturity, provided they were properly and carefully managed.
The greateft difficulty is to get the trees over, in order to be
tranfplanted in a right feafon, which is loft, by reafon that the
fhips for this voyage leave not Copenhagen till the middle of
May, at which time all trees are in bloom. However, with
proper care and caution they might be brought there, and made

* Mr. Anderfon tells us, that the earth will produce no fruit, chiefly on account
of the badnefs of the foil, the exceffive cold, and north winds. Experiments, he
fays, have often been made with various roots, but all to no purpofe.

L to

to thrive. Gardens are not only met with at Beſſeſted, the king's ſeat, but alſo at the ſeats of the biſhops, juſtices, and ſome of the lawyers; ſo that, there are gardens in every part of the iſland, and even in the moſt northern parts. At Skalholt, they have produced fine white cabbages. That the fruits of the earth do not attain the ſame perfection every where in all parts of this iſland, is not owing either to the ground or the air, but to the ignorance of thoſe, who neither properly prepare the ground, nor ſow in due ſeaſon. Here the fault lies, and it is not therefore ſurprizing, if things will not thrive. I have ſeen two gardens adjoining each other, but very different in their produce. That which was beſt ſituated to receive the ſun, and was ſheltered from the wind more than the other, was in the worſt condition : a remarkable inſtance, which ſhews plainly, that the ground in general may be cultivated in Iceland, though the winters are ſevere. I ſaw ſome cabbage in a garden, the latter end of Autumn in 1750, which by being neglected, was run to ſeed. This ſeed was then perfectly ripe, but being left to itſelf, dropt off, and in the ſpring of 1751, a great number of young cabbages ſprung up all round from the fallen ſeed which had planted itſelf, although the winter happened to be a very ſevere one, and the ſeed as good as lay on the top of the ground in a very diſadvantageous part of the garden, where little or no ſun could come *. After ſo many inſtances, who can be under any doubt of this country's producing vegetables, or can ſay, that the earth will not bring forth any fruit?

CHAP. XXIV.

Concerning the cultivating of the land.

WHAT has been already ſaid of the earth, the air, and their properties, will determine partly the preſent ſubject; which is, whether the earth can be cultivated and made to produce corn †. The ground that will produce garden fruit,

* Mr. Anderſon ſays, they have often attempted to ſow turnips, and various other roots, but always in vain; for nothing could be brought to maturity.
† The ſame Author ſays, that the ground cannot be cultivated, ſo as to be made capable of producing corn.

I pre-

I prefume, will likewife produce corn. In ancient days, the far-mers cultivated the land, and fowed corn for their own ufe. This is beyond contradiction; the people relate it, and it has been handed down to them from generation to generation. Be-fides, among their old laws are feveral chapters concerning ploughed lands, and land for fowing corn; by which it is alfo obfervable, that feveral difputes and law-fuits had hereupon ex-ifted. Thefe laws would certainly have never been made, un-lefs corn and other grain had been actually fown. Even to this day, fome pieces of land are met with, which are divided like corn-fields, and feem to have been ploughed, and properly tilled. Several farms, plains and fields, ftill bear the name of agre, or plough'd land; as for inftance, Akrekot and Akregierde, both adjoining Beffefted; Akrenefs, about 18 Englifh miles from it, and near it a place called Akrefield: all which ferve to confirm that the inhabitants formerly plowed and fowed their lands. How this moft effential part of hufbandry has happened to be fet afide, and how all the people have forgot to plow and fow, is not fo eafily accounted for, unlefs we charge it to that dreadful plague called fortedöd, which raging with fo much violence in the fourteenth century, almoft wafted this ifland of all its inhabi-tants, and left none able to till the land. By this means, agri-culture was entirely neglected and forgot, and fince that time, in the annals of this country, no mention is made of tilling, manuring, or cultivating any land. At prefent, there is a pro-fpect, with the bleffing of God, of reviving that part of hufban-dry; his Danifh majefty, having fent thither from Denmark and Norway able hufbandmen to introduce tillage, and to inftruct the inhabitants how to cultivate and improve their land. If all the land in Iceland was tilled that is fit for this purpofe, more ara-ble land would be found than in all Seeland and Fyen together. There is no occafion to take any trouble with thofe lands that are ftony and fandy. The other grounds which have refted now fome hundred years are fufficient, and they ftand in no need of any manure, though if they did, manure is not wanting; but I am very certain, if the ground is properly managed, it will produce excellent grain without any manure. In like manner,

I   I am

I am not of opinion, that the fummer, or warm weather, is of too fhort continuance to bring any thing to maturity. If the warm weather continues long enough to bring moft things wanted in a kitchen garden to proper maturity and perfection, and afterwards to feed, there is no doubt of the fame being long enough alfo to produce grain, which by the annals of the country we find has been. One need only remark, how very quick the grafs grows here, and as I before obferved, how in fome places it runs up in the fpace of 12 or 14 days two foot high *. The heat of the fun operates better than in more fouthern climates, and promotes vegetation in a ftronger degree ; for whatever is fowed, though later than in the countries more to the fouth, the fame ftill ripens in feafon, and even in colder climates than Iceland. In Lapland, where it is much colder, they fow, reap and gather in their harveft, all in the fpace of fix or feven weeks. The reverend Mr. Högeftröm gives an account in the memoirs of the Royal Society of Sweden, of rye in the fpace of 66, and corn in 58 days fown, and grown to perfect ripenefs. Why fhould not the fame happen in Iceland, where the fummers are both warmer and longer than in Lapland, which is proved by meteorological obfervations made in both places. In fhort, nothing but experience fhall ever make me believe the contrary. It is very probable, the feed may not profper every year alike, which fometimes happens in moft countries †. Iceland at prefent, muft be fupplied by other countries with meal, flour, and bread, great quantities of which are annually imported. Each harbour is furnifhed with, according to the number of the neighbouring inhabitants, from 300 to 600 tun of meal, befides bifcuit, of which they generally are provided with one third, in proportion to the quantity of flour or meal. The inhabitants purchafe according to their abilities, and fome ftock themfelves fo well, that they are never in want of bread all

---

* Mr. Anderfon fays, that no corn can grow in this ifland ; for if even the inhabitants were to put themfelves to the labour and pains of removing and gathering up all the ftones fcattered about on the ground, and of cultivating and manuring it, the fummer, or warm weather is of fo fhort a duration, that nothing can be brought to proper maturity.

† The fame Author repeats here again as another reafon, why the earth will not bring forth fruit, and this is, becaufe every where it is impregnated with fulphur.

the

the year round. Thofe that have it not in their power to do the like, muſt make other ſhifts; but it cannot be ſaid of any of them, that they know not what bread is. In the diſtrict of Skaftefield grows a ſort of wild corn, of which the inhabitants make bread, and though growing wild, it is in every reſpect as good as the Daniſh; nay, they will not exchange it for the foreign that is imported. This grows in ſand, and the ſeed that drops off ſows itſelf, and produces new corn regularly every year. The ſtraw, which is very good, they uſe to thatch their houſes with. This ſerves alſo for a proof, that corn may grow there, and that it will attain to a proper maturity. At leaſt they may ſow the ſeed that grows wild in every part of the iſland, this very ſeed, in all probability, being the relics of what they formerly ſowed their ground with.

C H A P. XXV.

Concerning ſea-weeds, and vegetables of the ocean.

THERE is a weed or vegetable that grows in the ſea, called *Alga-marina Saccharifera,* and by the Icelanders *Sol.* This the cattle are very fond of, and the ſheep alſo greedy after it, are often loſt by going too far out from the land at low water. It is very nouriſhing and fattens them, and the people alſo fond of it, gather and uſe it for their own eating, and ſell it to thoſe that dwell in the interior parts, where it bears half the price of dry fiſh. Hence it may be concluded, that as it is a thing the natives are fond of, they do not eat it out of ſcarcity or neceſſity. On the contrary, they always chooſe to have ſome of it by them. It is alſo very wholſome food, and it may be ſaid, that in this one particular, the ocean imparts a great bleſſing to this land. For a deſcription at large of this weed or vegetable, I will refer my readers to a diſſertation publiſhed by Mr. Biarne Poulſon an Icelander, and ſtudent in phyſic, concerning the *Alga marina Saccharifera* *. Beſides this

* Mr. Anderſon ſays, that he could not be informed of any other ſea-weed than the *Alga marina,* which both freſh and dry, for want of hay, they give their cattle. It fattens thems but makes the meat very nauſeous. In time of diſtreſs, the people alſo uſe it for food.

vege-

vegetable of the ocean, there are many other fea-weeds and herbs, which the fheep and cattle run greedily in queft of, though they have good grafs. Moft likely it is the falt tafte in all thefe weeds, that makes them fo palatable. The natives have peculiar names for the many fea-weeds and herbs found here, which is a fcience alone in itfelf. Coral is fometimes found, but few are curious enough to fearch for it. When it appears, it is fo chiefly by accident, as when fifhing hooks happen to catch hold of any. It were to be wifhed, that fome would think it worth their while to inftitute a coral fifhery. Since the above-mentioned ftudent in phyfic has began and given a treatife on one herb or weed, he may probably purfue fo laudable an undertaking, more efpecially as he now is there, and maintained at the king's expence for fome fuch purpofe, or to make a general collection of curious and extraordinary things *.

C H A P. XXVI.

Whether there are wild beafts in this ifland.

BEARS are fometimes feen there, but they come from Greenland on the floating ice, and are not native but foreign guefts, and fuch as the inhabitants do not choofe to naturalize among them †. Therefore fo foon as a bear is feen to fet foot on land, or his track is noticed, they ceafe not in their purfuit, till they have found and deftroyed him, without much ceremony. Thofe that live along the coaft have a fharp look out in winter and fpring, to fee whether the floating ice brings any bears ‡. They are likewife careful to furvey the fnow for the footfteps of that animal; and if they difcover any, one man alone is not afraid to purfue, attack, and kill him, and that generally with a gun, though many ufe fpears. In the northern diftrict, near Langenefs, where bears often come afhore, there lived an

---

* Mr. Anderfon declares, it is a pity that botanifts, efpecially Germans, have not attempted to collect and defcribe the fea-weeds and herbs that are here found in great abundance and variety.
† The fame Author afferts, that no kind of wild beafts, either noble or ignoble, or beafts of prey, are here met with but the fox.
‡ He alfo fays, that as foon as they difcover the footfteps of a bear, they affemble like a little army, and leave not off their purfuit till they have deftroyed him.

old

old man but lately dead, who had killed more than twenty in his time, and though a good markſman, always made uſe of a ſpear. He was greatly delighted when he ſaw a bear, and would purſue him alone, with no other armour than his ſpear, and never failed of victory, by charging him in front, and running the ſpear into his breaſt. This man did not degenerate from his ancient fore-fathers, the valiant Norwegians; nor did he want to raiſe an army to defeat a bear. If a bear unawares comes upon a man, who is not uſed to ſuch an encounter, or has not power to reſiſt, the bear may very likely fall upon him; but the natives here know pretty well how to get out of the way, by throwing ſomething at him to amuſe him. A glove is very proper for this purpoſe; for he will not ſtir till he has turned even every finger of it inſide out; and as they are not very dextrous with their paws, this takes up ſome time, and in the mean while the perſon makes off. It once happened in the northern diſtrict, that a perſon was killed by one of them; but the Icelanders are uſually very vigilant that none ſhould ſettle among them, chiefly on account of their cattle. Beſides, there is a reward for the hide, which muſt be delivered to the juſtice of the peace for the king. The Greenland bear ſkins are counted the fineſt and beſt that are, being white, grey, brown, and ſpotted.

C H A P. XXVII.

Concerning the Fox.

FOXES are the only wild beaſts in Iceland, and of them there is great ſtore *. They are generally of a dark red colour, (as the Icelanders call it) whereof are alſo a great many of the ſheep. This is the common colour of foxes in Norway and Denmark. The black ones, which are very ſcarce, are not natives of Iceland, but ſometimes are driven hither on flakes of ice. There are many white, and but very few grey. Thoſe that are white are ſo always, and don't change their co-

---

* Mr. Anderſon ſays, that the foxes in this country are never red; a few are black, and the reſt grey in the ſummer, and white in winter.

four

lour either winter or summer, which I myself can witness: neither do those of other colours suffer any considerable change, except when they cast their coat, at which time every creature differs in its appearance, a thing common and known by all. They use a kind of gin to catch them in, which they call a fox-shear; but more frequently destroy them by dragging the stinking carcass of a dead horse a good way about, which they leave on some field *. The smell invites numbers together to feed on the carrion, near which the people stand prepared to shoot them, and thus destroy a great many at once. It was also customary with them to dig deep holes, and make traps for them, in the manner of the wolf-traps in Norway; but this way they have quite left off †. Foxbane they make no great use of, not having the ingredients in their country, even the honey, that is used therein they must import, which makes the drug too expensive for them. These several ways they endeavour to destroy that hurtful animal the fox, that often robs them of a great many of their sheep.

C H A P. XXVIII.

Concerning horses.

THE horses are properly of the Norwegian breed, their sires being imported from that country, though parheps some of them came from Scotland, the Icelanders in ancient times, having carried on with that people a considerable trade. From them a great many Iceland words were introduced in the English, which I could not find out the derivation of, till I became acquainted with the Iceland language. The horses are not all equally small, a great many being large, and all in general very strong, lively, and brisk. They are the tamest creatures I ever met with. Some of the stone-horses are very mettlesome, as they usually are in most places ‡. The horses that are

* Mr. Anderson says, that they are very industrious in catching foxes in nets and traps, much like a taylor's shears, and rather this way, than by shooting at them, out of a natural aversion to fire arms.

† Bishop Pontoppidan, in his natural history of Norway, describes the wolf-traps used there.

‡ Mr. Anderson says, that the horses in Iceland, are extremely vicious and untractable.

set

fet apart for labour in the fummer, are kept out all the year round, and never come into any ftable *. They break the ice, and fcrape it away with their hoofs, till they get at the ground for fomething to nourifh them. The faddle horfes are kept in a ftable during the whole winter. Their fuperfluous horfes they mark, and afterwards turn out into the mountains, and there let them run for years together. Whenever they want them, they are obliged to catch them in a fnare; for they are entirely wild. A great many foal in the mountains, but the owners watch the time, and take care to mark the young foals. Among thefe wild horfes are fome very fierce and formidable ftone-horfes, who refolutely defend their own feraglio. Before they are caught and tamed, they will fly at the people that ride on the backs of other horfes to take them, and they often kill young ftone-horfes out of jealoufy. If they tame thefe horfes when they are about five or fix years old, they turn out very fine, keep their fat, and are never fenfible of any cold weather. The horfes kept entirely for labour, and out all the year round, are exceffive hardy, and very ftrong. In the winter they have longer and thicker hair, which helps them to bear the cold better, but towards fummer they get a new coat, and are very fmooth and handfome.

C H A P. XXIX.

Concerning the fheep.

THE fheep in general are as big as in Norway, Sweden, and Denmark, and I found them much alike in fize in all the parts of Iceland I travelled through. At Skaftefield they let the weather-fheep run about the mountains, all the year round, without ever houfing them; but fuch as give milk, they keep within in fevere weather. This cuftom is not univerfal all over the ifland, for eaftward and northward, at Arnefs and Borgefiorrs, and indeed in moft places, where they make it their bufinefs to breed cattle, all their fheep, mares, and cows, are houfed every night, and in fevere weather kept in all day, and at no time ever turn'd out in the fnow. Every farmer is

---

* Mr. Anderfon fays, that the horfes are kept to grafs, and expofed to all weathers all the year round.

pro-

provided with ftables and folds fufficient for his ftock of fheep, in the midft of which is a manger for hay *. I have feen four or five fuch fheep-folds to each farm, where they keep feperate the lambs, the weathers, and the fheep. At Guld-bringe, and a few other places, where they keep hardly any fheep, they have no fheep-folds; neither do I think they have any great occafion for them: for the two winters I was there, the cold was not too great for the fheep to be out during the whole winter, except three or four weeks in each, at which time fome of the farmers, more tender than others, took the lambs into their houfes, and fed them; becaufe the lambs under a year cannot bear the cold fo well as the old fheep, whofe backs are better covered to keep it out. There are caves and holes in the mountains capable of fheltering 100 or more fheep, where they very cordially retreat in bad weather. Thefe holes are in fuch mountains as have formerly burned, and are of infinite fervice to them both winter and fummer; in the winter for fhelter, and in the fummer for very good pafture, which they find in plenty all about †. No inconveniency is apprehend-ed from this their abode, except the treachery of their mortal enemy the fox, who harbours or lurks generally in thofe places, on account of the many holes and apertures in the rocks, and to pick up a nice fat bit among the fheep. If they happen to be out in frofty weather, they can make fhift to fcrape away the frozen fnow and ice, to get at the grafs underneath ‡. As for mofs, they never eat any, and I never heard but that there was always grafs enough upon the ground to fatisfy the fheep. Though they have folds or houfing for their fheep, where they keep them in the winter, yet when there is not much fnow, and the weather is fine and fair, they generally turn them out, partly to refrefh

---

* Mr. Anderfon fays, the fheep are very fmall, and are put to as great hardfhips as the horfes; for they never are taken in, but fuffered to be out in all weathers all the year round; their chief fhelter, if any, being under the rocks, and in caves and holes.

† According to the fame Author, the fheep always in winter keep clofe by the horfes, and continually follow them, becaufe in frofty weather they cannot with their feet break through the ice and fnow; but when the horfes have broke the way, they then can make fhift to get at a little mofs, (which the horfes leave) for their nourifhment.

‡ He alfo afferts, that the fheep have been feen through hunger and diftrefs, to eat of the horfes tails.

them,

them, and partly to fave provender at home, a good deal of the latter being required for 4 or 500 fheep belonging to one man. If it happens, when out, that fuddenly bad weather fhould come, together with ftorms of hail and fnow, they may fome-times be driven by the wind down to the fea-fide, and many of them may perifh *. Nay, I have feen even in fummer a flock of fheep carried away by a ftorm 60 or 70 Englifh miles. In the winter they may be alfo catched in heavy fhowers of fnow, and buried in it, efpecially as they generally feek the valleys at that time, and they may poffibly be two or three yards under the fnow, and loft for feveral days, till the weather admits their owners to feek after and releafe them †. In order to find them, they look out for a hole in the fnow, which indicates that the fox has been there. By his fcent he can find them out better than the people can with all their fagacity. The fheep are often refcued without any hurt. Sometimes they have been fcrouged and crufhed by the heavy weight of fnow upon them, but this happens according to the fituation of their place of refuge ‡. Sometimes they happily get to a cave, where they are well fe-cured, but it is a general rule with the Icelanders, to keep them within when they fufpeft any fuch weather. When the fheep are thus buried in the fnow, and are obliged to ftand a few days under it, they are often fo pinched with hunger, that they eat the wool off from one another's backs, which they make fhift of for fubfiftence, till their deliverance. All fheep will not do this : fome do, and get fuch a habit of it, that ever after they follow the fame practice ; but as foon as the proprietor obferves it, he kills them out of the way, on one fide, to prevent their be-coming fickly, and on the other, the fpoiling of the coat of the reft, whereof, if ftripped, they cannot bear the cold fo well.

* Mr. Anderfon fays, that when it both fnows and blows hard, the fheep have been carried before the wind from the mountains down to the fea, where they have perifhed.

† He again fays, that when heavy fnow falls, they are fometimes buried in it, and generally creep together, and with their heads clofe to one another, to let the fnow fall upon their backs ; but fometimes are fo frozen together, that they cannot be feparated.

‡ His opinion is, that from fuch a flock of fheep, a warm effluvium arifes, which opens a hole in the center of them like a chimney, whereby they are found out.

Young

Young colts and calves have often the habit of laying hold of the horses tails, and nibbling them, which will, as well as the wool in the sheep, gather up in balls as big as a walnut, and lie in the stomach undigefted. In the south parts they do not tend the sheep so well as in the north country, which there, is their principal concern. They seldom house them in these southern diftricts, by reason of the snows annoying them but little ; which according to my own obfervations, I never remarked above a foot deep at a time. They keep no shepherds to watch them, but to the eaftward, and in the north they do, whose sole occupation it is to give attendance, with a horse or two allowed them, and a couple of dogs trained up for this purpose. In the summer these shepherds take care of the cows, and in the winter, if the weather be fine, they turn out all the cattle, and at night drive them home again. The south inhabitants think this not worth their while, because they keep but few, though some farmers among them have from 100 to 500 sheep, befides oxen, cows, horses and mares. But as this ifland is very large, it is natural to think, that in places very remote, their oeconomy muft be very different. One, who has only been in the south, muft give as poor and as contemptible an account of their manner of keeping and breeding sheep and other cattle, as one who had only been in the north, of the Iceland fishing and fisheries. Both would conceive a very wrong idea of the ifland, and confequently muft give as indifferent a defcription, as many have already done, by only touching at particular places. The wool of these sheep is of different finenefs and goodnefs, as I apprehend it is every where. When forted and prepared, they make tolerable good cloth of it : but exclufive of the wool, God in his goodnefs, has provided these animals with an extraordinary coat, the better to endure the feverity of the climate. For this purpofe there grows a very coarse wool much longer, extending over, and covering the other wool. This the Icelanders call tog, which when mix'd with the other wool, it appears very coarse, but when carefully picked away, is not fo very coarfe, but that it makes very good woollen ftuff. The coarse they spin thread of, which is very ftrong, and is commonly ufed to few with. It is not always feparated, when brought to market,

2   ket,

ket, to be fold to the merchant; and as before obferved, it appears in that condition, extremely coarfe and rough. Their manner alfo of fheering it, renders it worfe to appearance; for they never cut it till the fkin is flead off the fheep, which they lay on their knees, and fcrape the wool off with a knife, by which means a deal of dirt and filth is at the fame time fcraped and rolled up with it. In the fpring of the year, towards the beginning of the warm weather, the wool falling off of itfelf, they watch and keep the fheep nearer home, that they fhould not lofe the wool. When it is quite ready to fall, the people pull it off quite clean, and afterwards fend them adrift. By degrees they get a new coat again before the cold weather comes in [*]. I have before obferved, that the fheep, commonly fpeaking, are kept near the houfes in the winter, when the weather is fevere; that a fhepherd is appointed to watch them, and that in the time of milking them, they never turn them out in the mountains, except where fome have feler or hutts to live in, and to houfe the fheep and cattle in the plains that lie between the mountains in the heart of the ifland [+]. Among thefe fhepherds, fome are fo expert, that at one view in a flock of two or 300, they can tell whether any of their fheep are miffing, which are, and what ftrange ones may be among them. They have a couple of dogs taught on purpofe to keep them together, and to drive them wherever they pleafe. They make ufe of no horn, or any other fignal than a hallow, which both dogs and fheep have learned to underftand, and in this manner they manage them, that every man may eafily mufter all his own fheep together, without much lofs of time. When the merchants at the meat

[*] Mr. Anderfon fays, the fheep drop their coat about the middle of the fummer, and that the outfide coarfe wool ferves to preferve them from the extreme feverity of the weather and piercing cold. But in order to fave the wool at the time they caft it, they are obliged to hunt and bring them together. For this purpofe, the huntfman going to the top of a hill with his dogs, and founding a fignal with his horn, the dogs feparate, and drive the fheep together from all corners into a pen, which is narrow at the entrance, but wide at the farther end, to prevent their flipping out again. At the time they kill their weather-fheep for victualling the fhipping, which lie in the meat harbour ready to take in their cargo, they are obliged to drive them together in the fame manner, which is done in the prefence of judges, to prevent the difputes that may arife about any one's claiming another's property; and as they are all inter-mixed, every one may go to the pen, and claim his fheep by his own mark.

[+] Bifhop Pontoppidan, in his natural hiftory of Norway, defcribes the places they call Seler.

or flaughter harbour, want to buy up any quantity, they give notice fome time before, upon which one man from each farm in the parifh or diftrict they intend to buy of, meet together on an appointed day, to go to the mountains and look for their fheep. When arrived at the place of deftination, the dogs collect all the fheep in one flock, and fence them in, perhaps to the amount of 8 or 10,000. All the fheep of the diftrict being thus gathered together, and fenced in, each farmer picks out his own fheep by the mark he has put upon them, and pens them up. As foon as each has his compleat number, they draught out as many as they chufe to fell. This is their way of collecting their fheep, which they do two or three times a year, fo that thofe which efcape the firft time, they get the fecond or third, and by this means each perfon mufters together his own fheep before the winter, in order to bring them home and houfe them. This cuftom they call in their language Saude-ret, which is as much as to fay to gather the fheep, that each man may pick out his own by his mark. No difpute can likely arife; for they put a very diftinct mark upon them, and each farmer in the diftrict is well acquainted with another's mark. The affair is carried on very peaceably among themfelves, though fometimes they have judges and juftices to decide differences, who likewife have their fheep there, but on their own account never appear in any other character than as farmers or proprietors of land in the diftrict. Some of the fheep have four horns, and fometimes befides them a little one, which may be called a fifth *: but thefe being rather looked upon as curiofities, are ufually fent to Copenhagen for prefents. It cannot be faid that they are common or all fo; for in a flock of 500, fcarce fix can be found with four horns, and fewer with five. As for more than five, I never faw nor heard of any fuch. A particular friend, who had a large flock of fheep, declared to me, he never faw any with more than five; and among all his flocks, he never had more than fix at a time with four, and very rarely any with five †. One third

---

* Mr. Anderfon fays, the fheep and rams have large curled horns, and generally more than four; fome have even eight, and frequently one in the middle of their forehead. On the contrary, the cattle, commonly called horned cattle, have here no horns at all.

† The fame Author fays, that the fheep in general have horns.

of

of the fheep here in general are without horns: even rams fometimes, and weathers, which ufually have larger horns than the
fheep. Two horns is what is common here, as in moft other
countries. Among the many thoufand fheep delivered every
year to the trading towns, very few have more than two
horns. A fheep with more horns bears a better price, and this
chiefly out of curiofity, and for the fake of rarity. Cows and
bullocks have horns, though fome have none; but northward
there are far more cows and fteers with, than without horns *.
I before obferved, that in moft parts of the ifland, the farmers make it their chief bufinefs to breed fheep, except in the
diftrict of Guldbringe, and I think they take a great deal of
pains to rear them all over the ifland †. Whilft the lambs fuck
their dams, they keep them at home, but when weaned, they
fend them adrift, yet towards winter drive them home again.
As the rams are let to run about among the fheep, to prevent un-
feafonable leaping, they tie a cloth under their bellies, which is
taken off towards Chriftmas. A great many fine young lamb-
fkins are exported from hence; for the people kill a great many
for their own eating, and many die by accidents; but few are
deftroyed by birds of prey, being watched when they are
young ‡.

C H A P. XXX.

Concerning goats.

I HAVE before obferved, that at Thingöe, in the northern
diftrict, and at Mule and Borgefiord, are confiderable woods,
but chiefly in the firft place, and that there are in feveral places
little thickets, bufhes, fhrubs, and heath enough, confequently
no want of fuftenance for goats in this country. In fome places
are great numbers, particularly in the north diftrict, where I may
fay, there is three times the number of goats to fheep §. Eaft-

---

* Mr. Anderfon fays that the cows and fteers in Iceland have no horns.
† The fame Author fays in fome places their greateft trade is with fheep, and there
the farmers take more care of them, and turn only the weathers into the mountains.
‡ He alfo fays the ravens deftroy many of the young lambs.
§ His opinion is, that they cannot keep goats in Iceland for want of food for them,
which confifts of the young leaves of trees.

ward

ward I have met with them alfo; they thrive very well, and yield great ftore of milk.

CHAP. XXXI.

Concerning cows and bullocks.

THE cattle in Iceland, both cows and bullocks, are as fine as any I have met with in Denmark. The cows yield a great deal of milk, I mean thofe of the better fort; for there is a difference here in cattle as well as in other countries *. Some cows yield 20 quarts of milk a day, others not above 10 or 12, and others lefs. This being a proper place to refume the fubject concerning their horns, I cannot help obferving, that I believe upon a juft average, that in the whole ifland there are confiderably more with horns than without. I allow, that to the fouth more are met with without horns; but northward, where the greateft number of cattle are bred, the horned have by far the majority. I before obferved, that fheep as well as faddle-horfes are kept in ftables in the winter, and there fed in proportion to the foregoing harveft, which if bad, their allowance muft necefarily be fcanty †. However, the farmer is careful to feed his cows in the beft manner he poffibly can, chiefly for the fake of the milk, a thing of too great confequence to be neglected. The cows are fed with hay, and fometimes with a fea-weed called fol, which they feem very fond of; but this weed is rather too expenfive to feed cattle with; becaufe the inhabitants eat it themfelves, and fell it for half the value of dried fifh. To the fouth in the right fifhing places, where the moft populous part of the country is, there is a neceffity of keeping many cows, though pafture-land is fcarce, to compenfate which, the inhabitants ufe their cows to eat fifh bones boiled foft, as alfo to drink the water they boil their fifh in. The cows in thefe parts,

---

* Mr. Anderfon fays, that the fineft cattle they have in Iceland are not bigger than the fmalleft in Germany, and obferves again, that in general they have no horns.

† The fame Author fays, that the cows only and young fteers have the good fortune to be fhelter'd in the winter, and fed, though very fparingly, with hay, which cofts the inhabitants a great deal of trouble and pains to get; when hay is wanting, he adds, that they then feed them with a dried fea-weed called fol.

by

by being accustomed to this manner of food, like it well, thrive upon it, and yield a deal of good milk.

C H A P. XXXII.

Concerning their milk, curds and whey.

THE Icelanders are very fond of milk, and always eat it, either raw or boiled; but do not choose that sick people should eat it before boiled*. Their chief liquor for drinking is whey, which they prepare in a particular manner. They make their butter of sweet cream, and when the butter is churned enough, they pour off the butter-milk, warm it, and as it grows cold, put rennet into it to make it curdle. Then they strain it through a linen cloth; the curds they eat, and the whey they keep for their common drink; the older it grows, the sourer and clearer it becomes. They keep it till it is as sour as vinegar, and make use of it to pickle with, but when they drink it, they must mix water with it.

C H A P. XXXIII.

Concerning butter and cheese.

AS there is plenty of milk in this island, consequently there must be a great deal of butter, which is generally made of sweet cream. First, they strain this milk through a sieve, before they skim it, and when the butter is churned, they put it in tubs or firkins †. But when they send their butter from one place to another by horses, they generally lay it up in clean sheep-skins, it being more convenient for the horses to carry it so than in tubs; this they do all over the country. They never salt their butter, and even cannot bear the taste of any salt in it; this I say of the people in general, for some among them, that have travelled and been in Denmark, by learning to like salt-

---

* Mr. Anderson says, that milk is the Icelander's chief medicine, and is used by none but the sick, who take it just as it comes from the cow.

† The same Author says, that their butter is always full of hairs: for they never strain their milk through any sieve, and when the butter is made, they put it in sheep-skins sowed up like bags.

butter

butter, falt theirs. Salt being a fcarce commodity in the ifland, the people have ufed themfelves to eat it without, and the tafte is therefore more agreeable to them. What can be alledged againft cuftom, and who will difpute any one's palate? Their butter looks very well, and I could have eat it for the looks, if my nofe did not tell me, that it could not tafte well [*].

CHAP. XXXIV.

The manner of flaughtering their cattle, and curing the meat.

THEY fometimes knock their cattle on the head to kill them, and fometimes ftick them in the throat with a knife [†]. The meat is generally eaten frefh, becaufe they do not love falt provifions, and the reafon probably is, upon account of the fcarcity of falt, and their not being ufed to it. The en-trails made ufe of, they wafh very clean, in the fame man-ner as people of other nations. When they lay in their winter provifion, inftead of pickling, they hang it up to dry, or they fmoak it, by which means they preferve it from putrefaction, and have provifion all the winter round [‡]. Many can well af-ford to falt it, but do not, having no relifh for falt meat, and they thrive and do as well with their provifion after their manner as other countries after their own.

---

[*] Mr. Anderfon fays their butter looks green, black, and of all colours.

[†] The fame Author fays, that the Icelanders do not knock their cattle down when they are about killing them, prefuming that the blood ftagnates or penetrates into the flefh, and prevents its keeping. Their manner of flaughtering, according to him, is to thruft a thin penknife into their necks, and when the creature falls, to tie its legs with ropes, and afterwards to cut its throat, that all the blood may run out.

[‡] He alfo fays, that thofe that can afford it, and have a mind to live better than their neighbours, buy falt, and before the carcafs is quartered, make three or four deep gafhes in different parts, into which they put falt, thinking that it will per-vade the whole as much as is neceffary to preferve it, during the drying or fmoak-ing. The poorer fort foak it two or three times in fea-water, then hang it in the air, and afterwards in the chimney to be fmoaked.

CHAP.

C H A P. XXXV.

Concerning their hogs.

NOT many hogs are now feen in this ifland, though there is great reafon to believe, that in former days there have been many. In the northern diftrict a few are kept, which thrive very well. The old annals of the country prove, that the country was formerly ftocked with a confiderable number. I found an account in them of two hogs, a boar, and a fow, being brought over, when this ifland firft began to be peopled. By fome accident they were loft, and three years after, found in a valley up the mountains, where they encreafed to upwards of 100. The place to this day is called fwine-dale. This is a plain proof, that they will thrive and multiply here. Many places in the ifland ftill retaining the name of fwine, there is no room to doubt, but that they formerly were in great plenty. There is Swine-næs, Swine-vatne, and a church near it, called Swine-vatne church, Swine-fkarde, Swine-hage, and Swine-völlum. By a piece of ground at Akrekor, near Beffefted, it is very obvious, that the fame was formerly hedged in, and that a hutt ftood therein for the fwineherd, which fpot to this day is called Swine-akre. Hence it is evident, that hogs were formerly bred here, and that they can find food enough, and will thrive; but the chief reafon why the inhabitants do not ftill keep them, is becaufe they fpoil thofe grounds near their farms, which they call tuner; befides, they cannot afford to keep people on purpofe to watch them. They may alfo well difpenfe with them, having a fuperfluity of other animals neceffary for their fubfiftance *. Dogs and cats are in plenty; efpecially the former, which the fhepherds, and thofe that look after the cattle, break and ufe for this purpofe. The people here are never feen without a dog, and every farm has a large houfe dog or two. Cats are not quite fo plenty, though very ufeful among them to deftroy the abundance of mice.

* Mr. Anderfon fays, they cannot keep hogs for want of food for them, of which a fufficiency can neither be found in the fields nor houfes.

CHAP.

CHAP. XXXVI.

Concerning tame fowl.

HERE are common fowls, such as cocks, hens, chickens, ducks, pigeons, &c. the same as in other countries. Eastward, and where the wild corn grows, which is very good food for them, they are chiefly kept, as also by those whose circumstances enable them to lay in corn and peas. They endure very well the weather, especially in the south parts, where the winters can neither be called severe, nor of a very long continuance *. In the northern district, which is the coldest in the island, I have met with pigeons and fowls, and I hardly ever heard of any perishing of cold. Sometimes a hawk or falcon will snap up a hen or chicken, but this I believe, happens oftner in Denmark or Norway; because having a much greater plenty of both wild and tame fowl. The reason why tame fowl are not kept so much here as in Denmark, is chiefly owing to the expence of corn, peas, &c. which must be from thence imported †. Here is plenty of wild ducks, and at certain seasons of the year, eggs of wild fowl in greater quantities than the inhabitants can consume. It would therefore be a folly to keep tame fowl at a great expence, when such plenty of wild fowl may be had without any expence at all.

CHAP. XXXVII.

Concerning wild land-fowl.

HERE are all sorts of snipes, ouzels, and beccasines in abundance; but quails there are none in the island. Partridges are native as well as in Norway, and in great plenty. The inhabitants shoot them, and can always procure a sufficiency of them for sale. They are never catched alive, but by the people

* Mr. Anderson says, that there is no such thing as keeping pigeons, or other tame fowl here, on account of the long and severe cold, want of nourishment, and the many various birds of prey.
† The same Author says, a few of the richest inhabitants that love a nice bit, keep a couple of fowls, which they make shift to feed with chopt hay, and a little rye meal mix'd with water.

that

that catch the falcons, who ufe them for a lure, and they too meet with difficulties in catching them alive, becaufe thefe birds finding food almoft every where, are not therefore eafily decoyed into a fnare *. As the falcon-catchers cannot depend upon getting thefe birds, they always keep pigeons and chickens for the purpofe, which they would have no occafion to do, if thefe birds were eafily caught.

C H A P. XXXVIII.

Concerning birds of prey.

NO great variety of birds of prey is obferved here. There are eagles, falcons, fome fmall hawks, and ravens, of which laft are great numbers †. It were to be wifhed, that falcons were more plenty. Owls and kites there are none. But as each of thefe birds requires a feparate article, I fhall therein treat of them more particularly.

C H A P. XXXIX.

Concerning the eagle.

THE inhabitants are not acquainted with more than one fpecies of eagle, which by what I have feen, feems to me to be a large fort. I did not hear that they do much mifchief, by deftroying any of their animals; if they do, it muft chiefly be the young and tender lambs ‡. But as the people very carefully watch their fheep and lambs, there is not much for them in this refpect. I have often feen the eagle hovering over the fea-fide, where there is a little inlet or creek, and there catch the fifh that come into fhallow water. They alfo have a way of frightening the hawk and falcon from the prey they have made, and taking it from them; for as the eagle cannot with

* Mr. Anderfon fays, that their fineft wild fowl are fnipes, quails, and partridges, called ryper, and that they run more than they fly, and are therefore eafily catched.
† The fame Author fays, that birds of prey are here in fuch variety and abundance, as hardly can be defcribed; viz. large eagles, kites, hawks, falcons, owls, ravens, and many more that have names, and many without.
‡ He alfo afferts, that here are various fpecies of eagles, which do the inhabitants a deal of mifchief, by deftroying all the young animals they can lay hold of.

Q   fuch such agility dart upon a partridge, or other wild fowl, they make no scruple of robbing the hawk or falcon, who catch them very easily *.

C H A P. XL.

Concerning the hawk.

THERE is but one species of hawk known here. Those I have seen, are very small, and cannot be reckoned among the terrible birds of prey. They are also few in number, and seldom pursue any thing but small birds, such as sparrows, except now and then a young chicken happens to fall in their way. They are mostly catched on the masts of ships out at sea, where they straggle some times a vast way, and too far to get back.

C H A P. XLI.

Concerning the falcon.

HERE likewise is but one species of the falcon. The cocks are in general remarkably smaller than the hens, which makes them appear to those that do not know the difference like different species. Some are white, some half white and half grey, but they are all of the same kind, and sometimes in one and the same nest, a young one of each colour has been hatched. This the inhabitants have declared to me, and I dare say, there is hardly a falcon-nest in the island without being known; for every falcon-catcher in his district takes care to watch them close, and to place his nets pretty near the place where they build. In winter sometimes whole flights of falcons come over from Greenland, and are chiefly white. The Iceland falcons are eminently the best of any for sport. A Norwegian falcon, or one of any other country, cannot be used above two or three years, but those of this island will last ten or twelve years and upwards. They are superior in size to any, and are endowed with many extraordinary qualities. The king of Denmark sends every year a falconer, with a couple of attendants to Iceland, to buy up the

* Mr. Anderson relates, that eagles have carried off children four or five years old to their nests; but our author assures us, that this is mere romance, no such thing having ever been heard of in the country.

falcons.

falcons. They go to Beſſeſted, where the king's falcon-houſe is, but it is not their buſineſs to catch them; for in every diſtrict there is a certain number of people licenſed for this purpoſe. They are all native Icelanders, and get by it a pretty deal of money when they are ſucceſsful *. It is about Midſummer that the falcon-catchers bring what they have caught to Beſſeſted. They come on horſeback, holding a pole with another fixed a-croſs, on which ten or twelve, falcons will fit all capped: the pole they hold in their hand, and reſt it on the ſtirrup. The falconer's buſineſs is to examine them, to return thoſe that are not good, and ſend the reſt on board the ſhip, to take back with him to Copenhagen. To the perſons that bring them for ſale, a written teſtimony of their reſpective qualities is given, by vir-tue of which, they receive of the king's receiver-general, fifteen rixdollars for a white falcon, ten rixdollars for one half white, and a gratuity from two to four rixdollars to encourage them for their pains in this buſineſs †. For a grey falcon they had for-merly five rixdollars, but for ſeveral years paſt, they have had ſeven rixdollars for every one of this kind.

An account of the manner the Icelanders catch falcons.

They ſtrike two poſts into the ground, a little diſtance from each other; to the one they tie a partridge or pigeon, (or for want of either, a cock or a hen) by a ſmall line two or three yards long, that they may flutter about a little, and that the falcon may the ſooner obſerve them; to the leg of the partridge or pigeon they tie another ſtring, 100 yards long or more, which goes through a hole in the other poſt, in order to draw the bait to that poſt, where a net is fixed, like a fiſhing net, with a hoop in a ſemi-circle of ſix foot diameter. This being pulled down, it goes over and covers the poſt, for which purpoſe, there is ano-ther ſtring faſtened to the upper part of the hoop, which goes through the firſt poſt to which the bait is tied. Theſe two ſtrings the falcon-catcher has hold of, that he may pull the bait

---

* Mr. Anderſon ſays, the king of Denmark ſends every year a falconer and two ſervants to Iceland to catch falcons, and to bring thoſe that are good to Copenhagen.
† A rixdollar is about 3 s. 6 d. ſterling.

where he pleafes, as alfo the net over his prey. Thefe nets they fix near a neft, or where they fee a flight of falcons approach. As foon as the falcon fees the bait fluttering on the ground, he takes a few fweeps about in the air juft over the place, and looks about to fee if there be any danger; then he ftrikes with fuch violence, that he takes the bait's head off as clean as if cut off with a knife. The moment he has ftruck the bait, he generally flies up again, unlefs very hungry, to look about if any danger be at hand, or any thing to interrupt him in the enjoyment of his prey. In the mean time of his flying up, the falcon-catcher pulls the ftring and dead bait to the other poft clofe under the net, which the falcon not obferving, prefently darts to devour his prey, but the other ftring being pulled, he is catched in the net *. He is taken out with the greateft caution, for fear of breaking any of his feathers in the wing or tail, and has a cap clapped over his eyes. The falcon-catcher is generally hid behind fome ftones or bufhes, or elfe lies flat on the ground, 100 yards or more off, where even if the falcon fees him, he has no miftruft, being at fuch a diftance. When the falconers return to Denmark with their complement, they lay in as much frefh meat as they think they fhall have occafion for to feed them, and befides take fome live cattle and fheep with them to kill by the way. They generally lay in ftore for feven weeks, for fear the voyage fhould prove fo long; for they do not choofe to put in any where by the way, not even in Norway, except they are under a neceffity †. They moiften the meat with a little milk for them, but if fick, they mix oil and eggs with it, which prefently relieves them. They keep always the caps on, both aboard and on fhore. During the voyage, the falcons are kept between the decks, tied to poles, two rows of a fide, and thefe poles are covered with coarfe cloth, and ftuffed with ftraw, and lines are flung from one fide to the other pretty clofe, that

*Mr. Anderfon fays, the falcon is catched by a bird (taught on purpofe) in a cage, put near the place where the net is fixed, which bird can fee the falcon at an incredible diftance, and by a certain noife gives notice, whereupon the falcon-catcher, who conceals himfelf in a bufh, throws out a pigeon to flutter about, which as foon as the falcon efpies, he ftrikes down upon, and immediately the net is pulled over him.

† The fame Author fays, that in their paffage they put in wherever they can for frefh provifion.

they

they may have something to catch hold of, if the ship should be tossed about, or if any of them should overset, that they might fall soft, and not too low to receive damage. By this account it is plain, that the falcon is no terrible bird of prey, and that one need not pity the Icelanders, when they acquire for them some money, and only rob them of a few partridges, of which they have more than they know what to do with.

CHAP. XLII.

Concerning owls.

THERE are no owls of any kind in the whole island *.

CHAP. XLIII.

Concerning ravens.

THE ravens here are black, and have nothing peculiar to distinguish them from those of other countries. They keep about the houses and farms, and steal what they can. Sometimes they kill a young and tender lamb †. No crows, magpies, or any of the kind are seen here; but there are four or six forts of small birds, which I believe they have not in Denmark; and which, as they have nothing particular to characterize them, I shall omit speaking of.

CHAP. XLIV.

Concerning the shore, or coast-birds.

NOtwithstanding the vast quantity of birds about the shore, most people that live along the coast know them all, and have a name for every one: but in a general description of a

* Mr. Anderson says there are various species of owls in Iceland, as the cat-owl, the horn-owl, and the stone-owl. He likewise published a print of one catched in the farther part of Iceland, on a ship homeward bound from Greenland.

† The same Author says, it has been observed, that in some of the small islands, especially the uninhabited about the coast, a couple of old ravens will settle, and not suffering any other to come near them, will fight and drive all away that offer to come. Our author says, he could not be informed of any such thing, though he took much pains to come at the truth of it.

country,

country, it cannot be expected that a full account can be given
of every particular; much lefs when the ornitography alone of
Iceland could furnifh out matter for a large volume.   The few
cliffs and fmall iflands about the coaft, abound with all forts of
fea-birds, and look quite white, by being covered with their
dung.   Thefe birds in large flights will ftray out at fea 30 or
40 leagues; but I cannot fay that I have ever feen fuch vaft
flocks fo as to darken the fun *.   Along the coaft, where there are
high and fteep mountains for them to build in, the fhore is
covered with them; but it is not fo round the ifland: for moft
places being low and flat towards the fea, but few harbour in
them, except when the fhoals of herrings come in.   At that
time the birds follow to catch them, which gives the fifhing
people timely notice, and is an agreeable warning to them.   At
the fame time alfo, great numbers of cod and other fifh perfe-
fecute the herrings underneath, as the birds do from above.
Some of thefe fea-birds are here during a ftated time, others
wander up and down, fuch as the oufel, the wild-goofe, &c. and
others live perpetually in the high rocks and cliffs towards the fea,
and the fmall adjacent iflands and rocks, where they lay their
eggs, and hatch their young †.   It is the large quantity of fifh
thefe feas are ftocked with, that makes fuch flocks of birds to
harbour here, add to which, their fecurity in the high rocks for
their nefts, though they are not fo fecure, but people can get at
them, and take away their eggs, which fhall be related in its
proper place, to fhew that the people are more cunning than the
fox, for they can get where he cannot.   There is a fifh called
rödmave, which delights to be near the fhore in fhallow water.
The fea birds catch many of them, among others the fea-gull,
who eats only the entrails ‡.   The blackbird (as they call it in.

* Mr. Anderfon fays, there are fuch vaft flights of fea birds, that they darken the
fun 30 or 40 leagues out at fea, and that their number and variety is fo great, that
none of the inhabitants know them, much lefs have a name for them.

† The fame Author fays, the feweft part of thefe birds ftay there the winter, towards which feafon they generally go away, probably to fome warmer climate, and
return in the fpring.   He adds, that this ifland is very convenient for them, by
reafon of the high rocks and mountains, where they fecurely make their nefts and
hatch their young, undifturbed either by man or fox.

‡ He alfo fays, that the fea-gull catches a certain well tafted fifh called runmave,
a good deal like a karuffe, and brings it afhore, and only eats the liver.   To this he
adds, that the farmers teach their children to fcare away the gull from his prey as
foon as he has brought it afhore, which they take up and bring home.

Iceland)

Iceland) takes a great many, and only eats the liver; but sometimes he is catched, or hunted from his prey, and if they find
it fresh, will take it away. The young children catch this fish
in the shallow water among the stones, they also catch several in
nets, and with rods: for when they throw out their line for a
cod, they frequently get only a rödmave. In most parts they
take them with a spear, like an eel-spear; for they are chiefly
close to the ground in very shallow water, and in calm weather
vast quantities of them may be seen, the variety of red colours
which they have, distinguishing them from other fish. This
fish has a large head, and several thick scales like lumps upon
it: the belly is quite red, from whence the Icelander calls it
rödmave or red-belly.

C H A P. XLV.

Concerning the shore-birds that are fit to eat.

SWANS and wild-ducks, as some imagine, do not leave this
island in the winter *. During the summer, they resort
the fresh water rivers, and in winter, when the fresh waters are
frozen up, they come down to the sea and open waters, where
continually great flocks of both forts are seen, not by scores, but
by several hundreds together. In the spring they return to the
fresh waters, and there hatch their young. I never any where
met with more swans and wild-ducks than in Iceland. The
swan being the largest and most excellent bird, deserves to be en-
larged upon somewhat more than the rest, to shew the advan-
tages the Icelanders reap from it. The swan is a constant inha-
bitant of Iceland, and vast numbers of them keep in the fresh
rivers up the country, where they lay their eggs, and hatch their
young. The eggs are large and very good eating. The season
approaching when they cast their feathers, and cannot very well fly,
the people go to the fresh rivers, and hunt and kill them. The
breast of a young swan, when well dressed is exceeding nice; but
the excellent down and feathers they get by them, fetch a deal
of money. At all other times of the year, they shoot them, and

* Mr. Anderson says, that among the eatable and well tasted shore-birds, the swans,
geese, and ducks are the first in rank, and never fail to appear in the spring.

frequently

frequently kill feveral at a fhot, by reafon of the large flocks they affemble in.

CHAP. XLVI.

Concerning the wild geefe.

THE wild geefe are not conftantly here, but come in the fpring, and go away at the latter end of autumn. Here are five different fpecies of geefe, divided into the mar-goofe, the helfinger, and the grey-goofe. The mar-goofe is but a little bigger than a duck ; the helfinger is the largeft of all, and has the whiteft feathers. As for the grey-geefe, the Icelanders have a particular name for each, and the fole difference between them, confifts in that the bill and legs in the one are red ; in the other, yellow ; and in the third, black. In other refpects they are all grey, and very good eating. It is not certain, that all thofe that come in the fpring, ftay here and breed ; becaufe in the nor-thern parts of the ifland, they have been feen to fet off again in great flocks farther north ; fo that it is prefumed, they fome-times only ftop here to reft. However, they pay for ftopping ; for the country people fhoot as many of them as they can, though their exceffive fhynefs makes them not very eafy to be fhot at : for while fome of them are at reft, others are watching, and up-on the leaft alarm, all fly away. Thofe that ftay grow tamer, and eafier to be fhot ; but in general they are difficult to be got at. When they come, feveral hundreds of them appear in one flock *.

CHAP. XLVII.

Concerning wild ducks, and down-birds.

IN Iceland there are upwards of 10 different fpecies of wild-ducks, which the natives have names for. Six forts of them are fit to eat, and are well flavoured. All the different kinds in

---

* Mr. Anderfon relates, that when the wild geefe come, they reft in the eaftward part of the ifland, and are on their firft arrival fo fatigued, that at that time they may be knocked down by thoufands.

Denmark,

Denmark, are alfo here. The beft tafted are very fmall, their body being not bigger than a pigeon *. The Icelanders call them örteænder, or trout ducks; becaufe they generally harbour where trout are; but of this fort there are not fo many as of the others. All the ducks in general are fit for eating, thofe only excepted that have a fifhy tafte. They are of three forts, and may be eaten, their tafte, as fome have imagined, being neither rank nor ftrong †. The natives call them langviget, lunder and alker. Among the various fpecies of ducks, the down-bird may juftly have the preference. This bird is much efteemed for its fine foft downy feathers, which the inhabitants turn to great account. Their eggs are alfo very fine. The drake is as large as a goofe, and has a great many white feathers, but the duck not much bigger than that of the common fize, is of a dark brown, yet fomewhat lighter on the breaft. Numbers of them are met with all over the ifland, though the greater part abide to the weft, upon account of the feveral iflands they feem to delight in. The inhabitants make little iflands on purpofe to invite them, and by thus confulting their convenience, get a great many more to come and fettle, being very fenfible of the advantage they bring. They like beft to build in defolate and lonely iflands, and if well treated, will build among people, and even clofe to houfes; but in this cafe, if the people choofe to make them continue in this abode, they muft fend all their cattle and dogs at fome diftance up the country, and if they live on a little ifland, they muft fend all their cattle away to the main land. It is very rare, though I have feen it, that this bird builds on the main land; but the people have enticed them to it by tender ufage, and by keeping them from being difturbed. If they do not difturb them, they may go about among them, even while they fit upon their eggs, and they will not ftir. They will alfo bear to have the eggs taken away from them, perhaps once or twice, yet ftill will lay others, and hatch their young, and the next year come to the fame

* Mr. Anderfon fays, all their ducks have fuch a fifhy tafte, that none are fit for eating.

† He alfo fays, that the Icelanders are quite regardlefs of the tafte of birds; for whether taken in the rocks where they climb to catch them, or on the fands, all are thrown into the pot and dreffed, according to their fafhion, and fo eaten, their ftomachs being fo good as not eafily to be turned.

place,

place, and continue multiplying as long as they are well ufed. The advantage received from them, is in the down and eggs. When thefe birds build their neft, they pluck the down from their breaft for the eggs to lie on, and to keep them warm. They lay four eggs, as big as goofe eggs, and green; and when they have done laying this number, the people perhaps finding them, take them away, as alfo the down, and fo fpoil the neft. Notwithftanding, the ducks going to work again, pluck more down from their breaft, and lay other eggs: the people then come and take the down and eggs away a fecond time. Still patiently they go to work a third time, but the ducks having plucked themfelves bare before, the drakes now fupply the neft with down. The laft is therefore beft and whiteft, (for the drake is white, the duck brown on the breaft). She then lays her number of eggs over again; but if taken away, lays no more, nor ever builds a neft there, but looks out for another place the next year. For which reafon, a good oeconomift will take care and watch, that the third lay of eggs is not taken from them, and that they are fuffered to lie peaceably, and to hatch them. Then they may be certain, that the next feafon, fhe and her young will come there again, and inftead of one neft, will make two or three. When the young ones leave the neft with the old, the people gather the down a third time from the neft, and in this manner get two fets of eggs, and three parcels of down from each neft. Hence it may be judged, what vaft advantage they have by them, confidering how many thoufands build among them. Their eggs are as good as any hens eggs. The down they pluck off themfelves is much the fineft, though all the reft of their feathers are very good and ufeful *. The good oeconomift will not fuffer any of thefe birds to be fhot, or a gun to be fired near them, efpecially while they are building, for fear of frightening them away. In this manner they get great quan-

* Mr. Anderfon fays, the feathers that are pulled off when they are dead are of no ufe, becaufe they are fat, and putrify very foon. He adds, that when tho young ones fly out of the neft, the people who are upon the watch, go and take the down away. Bifhop Pontoppidan obferves the fame in his natural hiftory of Norway, where he fays they lay many eggs which are long, and of a dark green colour; and if a ftick a foot long is ftuck in the middle of the neft, they will continue laying till it is covered, that they may lie convenient, but this weakens the birds to fuch a degree, that they fometimes die.

titics

tities of down and eggs, without deftroying or hurting the birds. The down they export, and rather make a pecuniary advantage of, than ufe it to gratify their own eafe.

CHAP. XLVIII.

Concerning the diver or the plungeon.

WE have but one fort of thefe ducks called divers or plungeons. They are well tafted and fit to eat [*]. They are not very fifhy; for the Icelanders not liking any fowl that has a trainy or fifhy tafte, are under no neceffity of ufing that which is not good, amidft fuch plenty and variety.

CHAP. XLIX.

Concerning the lomen, or northern diver [†].

THE lomen or northern divers, much about the bignefs of a goofe, have a narrow bill and fmall wings, and grow very fat and heavy. Their legs ftanding very much behind, they walk with as much difficulty as they fly, on account of their fmall wings and heavy body. They make a frightful noife, and are far from a pleafing bird to look at; at leaft I could fee no beauty in them. Neither their flefh nor eggs are fit to eat. This bird is unmolefted; for the people give themfelves no trouble to look after its neft or brood [‡]. They build in remote places near frefh water, that they may reach to drink without moving from their eggs, or if they fhould want to move, that they might do it the more conveniently, by reafon of their being fuch bad walkers and fliers. As this bird alfo does not build about the fea-fhore, it is improperly called a fhore-bird.

[*] Mr. Anderfon fays, fome of the divers or plungeons are fit to eat, but many not.
[†] In the Orkneys they call this bird embergoofe.
[‡] Mr. Anderfon relates, that the Icelanders having never been able to difcover where the northern divers build, pretend that they hatch their young under their wings.

CHAP.

C H A P. L.

Concerning the geir or vulture.

THE vulture-rocks, called alſo bird-rocks, lie beyond Rei-kenes, in the ſouth diſtrict, about ſix or eight leagues weſt of this place. On theſe cliffs and rocks are a great many vultures, which beſides harbour in other parts of the iſland. The inhabitants at a certain ſeaſon go to theſe iſlands, though the expedition is very dangerous, to ſeek after the eggs of this bird, of which, they bring home a cargo in a boat big enough for eight men to row. The danger and difficulty conſiſts in get-ting aſhore near theſe cliffs which lie ſix or eight leagues out at ſea, where the water generally runs ſo high, that if the boat be not very carefully managed, it runs the riſque of being daſhed to pieces againſt the rocks by the violence of the waves *. Though there are not ſo many of theſe birds as of other ſea-birds, yet they are not ſcarce. They are frequently ſeen, and thoſe that go to take their eggs from them ſee enough of them. The eggs are very large, and almoſt as big as oſtriches eggs.

C H A P. LI.

Concerning the ſhore-birds neſts.

IN the high and perpendicular cliffs near the ſea ſide, and in the cracks and holes, and where the rocks hang over the water, the ſea and ſhore birds build in incredible numbers. The inhabitants get at theſe places, notwithſtanding all the caution the birds take to hide their eggs, or to build in almoſt inacceſſi-ble places, and they plunder the neſts of their eggs and feathers. It being impoſſible for them to climb the rocks, by reaſon of many hanging conſiderably over the water, they therefore, in order to get at the birds and their neſts, thruſt out a long beam

---

* Mr. Anderſon ſays, that the geir or vulture is not often ſeen here, except on a few cliffs to the weſt, and that the Icelanders, naturally ſuperſtitious, have a notion that when this bird appears, it portends ſome extraordinary event. Of this he aſſures us his being told, that the year before the late king Frederic IV. died, there appeared ſeveral, and that none had been ſeen before for many years.

towards the top of the rock, which they faften at óne end to the ground, and at the other with a long rope that flides through a hole made in the beam. By this machine, they raife up, or let down the man that is to take the eggs, who, when he has got as many as he can carry away with him, gives a fignal for retiring *. In this manner they go on as long as eggs are to be found, or as long as they are able to hold out. The man that is let down has a pole with him, by which he pufhes himfelf out, or draws himfelf farther in, juft as he fees occafion. When the birds are attacked by thefe people, they fly away by thoufands, making a terrible noife and fhrieking. In the parts where thefe high cliffs are, the inhabitants have vaft benefit and advantage by the birds. Befides the eggs they take, they catch vaft numbers of the birds, many of which, as I before obferved, are very fine eating, and of the feathers they make a very good trade, exclufive of what they keep in the ifland for their own ufe. I have feen the people catching the birds in this manner, and muft confefs, that it is very dangerous work. Sometimes accidents happen through carelefsnefs, by the beams giving way, or by ufing a rope that is not ftrong enough. Thefe birds, though they build fo thick and clofe together in the rocks, and are fome thoufands in number, yet all find the fpot at once where they have built, never miftaking their neft, though fo like each other, as not in any refpect to be diftinguifhed.

C H A P. LII.

Concerning the fhore-birds eggs.

THE eggs of the fea and fhore-birds are of a greenifh colour with black or brown fpots. They have a thicker fhell than land birds, fo ordered, I fuppofe, by Providence : for as thefe birds are obliged to feek nourifhment at a very great diftance from the place where they build, and lay their eggs, and confequently are fometimes a long while abfent from their rooft, the thicknefs of the fhell muft preferve fo much longer the in-

---

* Mr. Anderfon fays, it is with the greateft danger of their lives that they climb the fteep and rugged rocks to get at thefe birds nefts.

ternal

ternal heat, and prevent the external cold from penetrating to deftroy the tender life within. Thefe eggs are for the better part well tafted. There is alfo a fmall bird here which the Icelanders call kreye, whofe eggs are extremely nice.

CHAP. LIII.

Concerning the vaft quantity of fhore-fifh.

TOO much cannot be faid of the great blefling which God has beftowed on this ifland, by the vaft quantities of fifh the fhores abound with all round the ifland, and the vaft variety, both large and fmall, for nourifhment and ufe. It is fuppofed thefe immenfe multitudes of fifh come from more northern parts to Iceland in their peregrination to the fouthern, though many proceed no farther, which is very reafonable to think; becaufe in fome parts of this ifland there is good fifhing all the year round, chiefly of fine fmall cod, which very probably are only the young of the larger fort, being in every refpect like them. The inhabitants relate by the obfervations they have made, that the codling goes three times round the whole ifland with the wind, and when gone the third time, are grown to a full fize, and become what is properly called the large cod. The cod that come in fhoals towards the fpring of the year, being much fatter and finer than thofe fifhed for at other times, there will be no improbability in fuppofing, that they have lain under the land all the winter. The people in particular remark the courfe the fifh take; they appear firft eaftward of the ifland, then fouthward, and afterwards about the great creek or bay between Reikenefs and Wefter Jokel. This creek is twenty or twenty-four leagues broad, and runs fixteen or twenty leagues up into the country. Here are their greateft fifheries, and from hence moft of the harbours to the fouth are fupplied, except the harbour of Grindevig. To this place alfo they come from all parts round to fifh, even from the northward in the fifhing feafon, which they call vertiden, and fometimes ftay the whole fummer and autumn a fifhing. More fhall be faid with regard to this place, in the chapter concerning the fifhing feafons.

CHAP.

C H A P. LIV.

Concerning the shore-fish, or such as in general keep along the coast.

AS in a general description of a country, a complete ich-thyology, or particular description of all the fish through-out the country cannot be expected; it is not my intention to make a voluminous work, which I know myself not qualified for, not having furnished myself with sufficient materials for such an undertaking, though I lived upwards of two years in the island. I shall therefore pursue what I chiefly intended, which is to give a brief account of the island, and to range every thing in proper order, to make every article intelligible, and convey a true idea of the place to my readers. I presume to say, that I know much more of the place than many, who have published their accounts of this island, according to very imperfect and false ideas, and consequently their publications, must have propagated the same, which I am very desirous to remove, hoping that this short treatise will have that effect, at least on those, who have not received too strong a prejudice from those false and erroneous accounts that have before been published.

C H A P. LV.

Concerning herrings.

HERRINGS come from the most northern parts, where they breed, and send forth vast colonies to all Europe at certain seasons. They return again to the north, and in that manner annually make their progressions. In passing by Iceland, they are usually driven by the whales and other large fish, as chaff before the wind, and sometimes they are chased into the bays and creeks of this island in such numbers, that a boat can hardly be rowed through them, and they well might be taken up by pails full; though this happens but seldom. The Icelanders do not apply themselves to herring fishing, having neither materials for it, nor knowledge how to cure the fish; add to which, their great scarcity of salt. It is therefore for these reasons that they

4 do

do not trouble themselves about taking more than they can make use of fresh. Very likely if they had salt sufficient, and understood how to cure them, the merchants would not take them off their hands, because they are not taxed; from whence one may conclude, that Iceland is not a proper place for herring-fishing, except when the above-mentioned extraordinary accident of their being driven into the creeks and bays in such excessive quantities happens *. Otherwise the Icelanders would no doubt have laid themselves out for herring-fishing, and their price would have been taxed as other fish are: for they are very sufficient for the undertaking, in respect to the number of hands that should be employed; neither are they so indigent in circumstances, as not to be able to manage a very considerable fishery, especially since the king has generously supplied them with a considerable quantity of necessary implements, which may put this and other fisheries upon a very good footing. What I mean by herrings, that do not appear in the creeks and harbours of this island in great shoals, unless by accident, are the fine large fat herrings fit for pickling †. At all other times a vast plenty of small young herrings like pilchards or sprats, arrive with the cod, which this fish feeds very agreeably on, as do also from above the birds, by whom they are snapt up. Together with these persecutors, the whale swallows them up in heaps, which has been often seen here; and once in particular, a whale pursuing his prey too greedily, run aground, and the tide setting out, left him helpless on the shore. The inhabitants soon gave him his quietus, and found in his belly upwards of 600 fine live cod, together with a great quantity of herrings, and some birds. These small herrings are of two forts; the one is called by the inhabitants sand-herrings, because they lie upon the sand banks in the sea about the coast, almost all the year round; they are often also found in the bellies of large fish when any are

* Mr. Anderson says, he knows very well, that all the creeks and harbours in Iceland abound with the finest and fattest herrings, and that if it was not for the scarcity of people, and their indigent circumstances, they would be able to carry on the greatest and most advantageous trade imaginable in this very one respect.

† He also says, there are many different species of herrings, but he never met with any who had been curious enough to make proper observations or remarks. He speaks of one fort eighteen inches long, and three or four inches broad, but our Author says he never heard of any such.

caught.

caught. The other are called the hairy herrings, becaufe they have a ftripe all along the back like hair, and when feen or found in the bellies of any fifh, the people are fure the cod is not far off, becaufe this fifh is only periodically about the ifland. Herrings, efpecially the large ones, are the beft bait to catch cod with, though not ufed by the Icelanders, becaufe they cannot always get them *. It is remarkable, that the cod and large herrings do not always come together, if they did, the people would fuffer greatly in their cod-fifhing. The large herrings refort not to this coaft every year, but the fmall fprat kind always attend the cod, and are their common food. The Icelanders catch none of thefe fmall herrings, being unprovided with nets for this purpofe, and depending principally on their cod-fifhery. It is a diverting fight to fee, when thefe fmall herrings come in fuch glutts on the coaft, how the birds by thoufands hover above, and like a dart ftrike down upon and catch them. This continually happens, whilft the fifh are making all the way they can to the coaft to get into the creeks and bays, though even there they become an eafier prey to the birds.

C H A P. LVI.

Concerning the cod.

THIS fifh, called by the Icelanders torfk or kabbelau, which names are fynonimous, is caught moftly about the fouth and weft parts of the ifland †. Northward and eaftward, they hardly catch enough for their own confumption, and are often obliged to have them from the fouth and weft quarters, where they buy them up dried, or fend their people there to fifh and cure them for their ufe. But the great quantities of flefh, train of whales, feals and cods, the down and feathers of the birds, and the wrought and unwrought wool of the fheep, afford fubfiftence to as many of the inhabitants as the fifhery does. In the right fifhing places,

* Mr. Anderfon fays, that the Greenland traders when they intend to catch cod, and are in want of a frefh herring for a bait, make ufe of an artificial one made of tin, which ferves as well as the natural one. Our Author fays he tried the fame experiment, but it did not anfwer; for they would rather lay hold of a bit of beef.
† Mr. Anderfon alfo fays, that cod is the chief food of the people of this ifland.

U   variety

variety of other fish is caught befides cod, which I fhall prefently make appear, and though not a merchantable commodity, they ftill are of great ufe for the food and fubfiftence
of the inhabitants.   In certain places up the country, are frefh
rivers and lakes, with great plenty of trout, and there the
people have no great occafion for the dried fea-fifh; for they dry
the frefh water fifh, and lay it up for ufe; and indeed dried
trout is very delicate eating.   They catch all their fifh with a
hook and line of fixty fathom length, and put for a bait eight
or ten mufcles on the hook *.   The mufcles here are very large
and fine, and full as large as any I ever faw in Holftein.   Very
feldom they make ufe of the gills of cod, rather chufing to take
a piece of another fifh.   Befides mufcles, they dig at low water a
black ugly worm out of the bottom of the fea, which they ufe
for a bait; as alfo the entrails of fhore-birds, and their raw
flefh, which is reckoned a very good bait.   All are not equally
lucky at fifhing: for when a parcel of boats have been together
on the fand-banks a fifhing, fome of them will go away full,
whilft others have got hardly any thing, though they ufe the
fame bait.   They have plenty of wild fowl at hand, if they find
the fame a good bait.   There is no law againft their ufing any
thing, and I am perfuaded they ufe what bait they like beft.
When the fifh come in great fhoals, it may be perceived on the
water, as alfo when they are purfued by the whale; for then
they are in great confufion, and are fometimes feen above the
water.   At that time they will not bite, and fcarce ever but
when they are quiet on the fand-banks in the fea, which the
people well know, becaufe they then bite, and are catched
apace †.   They likewife will bite, even fometimes at a hook
without any bait, if tinned and bright, when they come in
great heaps without being hunted in or fcared by the whale.

* Mr. Anderfon fays, that they catch all their fifh by angling, putting a bit of a
mufcle on for a bait, or fome of the gills of the cod they have catched; but they bite
beft at a bit of raw flefh of the birds while warm, or the heart of a fea-gull juft
fhot.   With fuch a bait one may catch twenty, while another with the bait they commonly ufe, will hardly catch one; but thofe artifices are forbid by the king, that one
might not have the advantage of the other.
† The fame Author avers, that when the fhoals of fifh come, the number is fo
prodigeous, that their fins appear above the water, and that they will bite at any
thing, even at the bare hook, without any bait at all.

They

They generally in this cafe keep very deep in the water. The right fifhing feafon, which is called by the Icelanders vertiden, begins the third of February, and lafts till the twelfth of May. At this time multitudes of the inhabitants come from the north and eaft, (in which parts no fifhing is carried on in that feafon) and fome of them continue here during the whole fummer a fifhing, before they return home to the north. Their feafon begins the twelfth of May, and lafts till the harveft is in *. They cannot begin before, on account of the floating ice that comes from Greenland ; fo that the fifhing feafons cannot be at one and the fame time throughout the ifland, though fometimes it happens, that after the twelfth of May, when the feafon ought to end in the fouth quarters, they get the moft fifh, and dry them, both for home confumption and exportation †. Though the feafon is over, if they have had but little fuccefs, their heart not failing them, they wait ftill longer, and are fometimes plentifully rewarded. They always fifh whilft any thing is to be got, and while the weather permits. They are out often night and day, fometimes in the deep, fometimes in the fhallows, and never mifs any convenient opportunity, efpecially from about the middle of April ; becaufe then the nights beginning to be very fhort, they can remain out the whole night, and it is light enough for them to go any where. Before that time they only fifh a days, and are generally out two hours before the fun rifes, and return home when it fets. But if they have not got their cargo, and find the weather promifes fair, they ftay all night, fo that they do not confine themfelves to any time, but make ufe of night or day in fome places, juft as it happens. In general, the fineft and moft delicate fifh are caught in forty, fifty, or a hundred fathom deep of water ; but it cannot from hence be inferred, that the fifh taken in the gulphs or near the fhore, are not fo fat and fine ; for when the fifh firft arrive, they are as fat and fine as any where in the deep waters. It is true, thy fall off fome time after ; but thofe far out at fea, and on the banks, keep up better

* Mr. Anderfon fays, the right fifhing feafon begins the fecond of February, and lafts till the firft of May ; for then it begins to be too warm to cure and make them fit for keeping.
† The fame Author fays they fifh in the gulphs and deep fea by day, but near fhore, or in eight or ten fathom water by night.

than

than thofe near fhore or in the creeks, where they probably do not meet with fuch nourifhment. The Icelanders cure their cod but one way, and when cured, they call it flat-fifh. It is exported to Copenhagen and Gluckftad, and is a fifh very well known, and as well tafted as any found or cured elfewhere. Weftward they hang them up to dry, and call them hang-fifh. They have houfes on purpofe to dry them, which are built of lathes, pretty wide afunder, for the air to draw through, and a covering to keep out the rain. To cure them this way, they flit open their backs, and run a pole through them, and then hang them up to dry. The flat-fifh have their bellies flit open, and are afterwards fpread out to dry. The hang-fifh are fomething cheaper than the flat-fifh, becaufe flat-fifh is the merchantable fort; and therefore there are a hundred flit and dried flat on the ground, to one that is hung. When the fifhermen land with their cod, they lay them out along the fhore, cut off their heads, flit open their bellies, gut them, then flit them quite down, and take out the back-bone from the head down to three joints below the navel. This the men do themfelves. The foreman of the boat divides the fifh, and every one that went has his lot *. When they have flit them, and taken the back-bone out, they double them up, together again, and lay them one by one, if the weather pro-mifes fair the next day, to fpread them out to dry; but if the weather looks otherwife, they fpread the fifh out, and lay them one over the other, the fkin fide upwards, and fo let them lie a day and night; but take care not to let them lie too long fo for fear of fpoiling. The women have nothing to do in the affair, except fometimes, when fome of them may come to help their wearied hufbands. When they have prepared their fifh fo as to get it ready to lay out to dry, the next day they return home no doubt much fatigued after their days hard labour, to take reft and refrefhment, and have fome of their fineft fifh dreffed for themfelves and their families; but as they always catch other fifh with the cod, they rather choofe to eat them frefh, or if

---

* Mr. Anderfon fays, that when the men come afhore with the fifh, the women go down to the fea-fide, and begin to work upon them, by cutting their heads off, flitting and gutting them, &c. He calls them flit-fifh, becaufe they are flit open; but our author calls them flat-fifh, becaufe they are fpread flat on the ground to dry,

　　　　　　　　　　　　　　　　　　　　　. they

they boil a cod, they boil the head with it*. The heads they cut off they dry as well as the fish, and get a good price for them in the country. The bones that are taken out of the fish are used in some places for firing by the poor people, where there is a scarcity of fewel, as there generally is along the coast. They likewise use them, as has been before observed, to feed their cows and cattle with, by first softening them in boiling water. The livers they stow up in a vessel, and boil them all together to make train-oil. Brandy is a scarce commodity with them, and but few can afford it. That which is offered to them for sale, is seldom fit to drink after Easter. Thus they do not much care for that liquor; but if they could, as the fishing people in most countries, take a good dram before they go out, and have another when they come home, it would do them no harm, and perhaps, in a great measure, would allay the sense of the almost incredible hardships they suffer. They are sometimes eight or ten leagues out at sea before the day breaks, and all night long when it is light and fine weather. All this time they continue fishing with their long lines, without any victuals, or any refreshment but their common drink called fyre, (which I have already described). When they have rowed themselves back again with their cargo, sometimes with the greatest danger of their life, in tempestuous weather, their next care is to get ready their fish for drying, which being done, they must take a long walk to their respective habitations. After all this, it is reasonable to suppose, that they require rest and refreshment, and a good dram; but the last hardly one in a hundred has. The only thing they indulge themselves with at sea, beside their liquor, is tobacco, which they make use of three different ways, each according to his taste.

I will now give a short and circumstantial account of their manner of managing their flat-fish. When they have cut the head off, and slit open the belly, the entrails are taken out, then the fish is quite laid open, and the back-bone taken out, afterwards it is doubled up, or two are put together, the flesh part to each other. This is done when the weather is clear, and

* Mr. Anderson says, when they have done this work, the women carry home the cods heads to dress for their family; the bones they use for fewel, and the livers they save to boil oil out of; the men then go home, and indulge themselves with brandy according to their circumstances.

X

the air dry, that they may the next day spread the fish out upon the stones; but when the weather is damp, or a frost happens, they then lay them in little heaps upon one another, with
the skin upwards, and let them lie till the weather is fit for
drying, at which time they spread them out upon stones if they
can, but where they have no stones, along the coast, and this
they do the day after they arrive with them if the weather will
admit of it, for it makes the fish much better, though they generally receive no damage by lying three or four weeks in kase, as
they call it, which is in little heaps upon one another, provided
it is not very foggy or damp weather, or too hard a frost. Whilst
they lie to dry, the women go and turn them several times a day,
that both sides may imbibe equal portions of the sun and air.
In fine weather they will thoroughly dry in fourteen days, though
they generally take more time. When the fish is quite dry, they
are heaped up together upon the stones, and then will receive no
damage from any kind of weather *. Each lays his lot together,
and piles it up about as high as a man can reach; but when the
fish are brought to market from each district, they pile them then
as high as houses, or like great stacks of hay. They sell all
they can, without ever bringing them under roof; but what
they keep for their own consumption they lay up in their houses.
When the merchants have got them in stacks, and it threatens
wet weather, they cover them to keep off the rain, till they can
conveniently ship them, which they do as soon as possibly they
can. In sending them aboard, care is taken that they contract
no damp in the place they are deposited; the reason is, because
there is a great difference between their being packed down close
in a ship, and their standing in stacks, where the air draws
through, and dries them immediately after they have been moi-
stened. The hang-fish are prepared in the same manner as the
flat-fish, saving that they are slit down the back to run the pole
through, whereon they hang to dry in houses built for that purpose, as has been already described †. They also are hanged

* Mr. Anderson says the skin side is always turned upwards when they dry them,
for fear the rain should spoil the flesh, and if there happens to come a north wind, the
fish may be thoroughly dried in three days.
† The same Author says, that for the houses to dry fish in, they only raise four
walls of scraps of stone heaped on one another, without any thing to bind them together, and make it as open as they can for the wind to draw through, covering it
with boards and turf to keep out the rain.

up the day after they come from fea. Fifh is only cured in the weft after this manner, and not in every place, though moft people have a houfe to dry fifh in of other forts, where they only dry them in the air without the fun. The fifh dried along the fhore where no ftones are found, are laid upon the hard white fand, and not upon the bones of fifh. Dried in this manner, the fifh is whiter, and dries fafter than otherwife, becaufe the fun has more power to act and infinuate itfelf. It alfo will keep as long as any other, and the only accident it is liable to, is that it becomes fandy, and may for this reafon be rejected by the merchant *. It is the fine dry and clear air here that dries the fifh fo well. The days at this feafon are longer than in more fouthern countries, and the heat of the fun not fo piercing. They continue to dry fifh all the fummer, though in the midft of fummer they turn not out fo well. The great heat breeds maggots in, and fpoils them; the ftrong fmell alfo of the fifh attracts the flies, and I have feen them even in April, as thick as poffible about them. In the autumn the fifh will dry very well, if the weather does not turn out too wet †. The Danifh merchants in Iceland pickle feveral hundred cafks of cod a year, which they export to Copenhagen, befides curing a great deal of klip-fifh. The inhabitants do the fame with regard to the klip-fifh, but it is generally for their own ufe, or to difpofe of at home, becaufe they know not how to cure it well enough, to make it anfwerable for a foreign market. At beft, they cure not much this way, upon account of the expence of falt, and the fifh not fetching more than the dried, even exclufive of the falt and cafks, it cofts much more trouble than the dried, which

* Mr. Anderfon fays, that the fifh dried on ftones is much preferable to that dried on the fand, being firmer, whiter, and keeping longer; whereas that dried on the fand, being laid upon the bones taken out of the fifh for want of ftones, changes colour, and will not keep fo well.

† The fame Author fays, it is very furprifing how fuch large fat fifh can be cured in the Iceland manner without falt, and piled up in the open air without corrupting; but on the contrary, be fo found as to keep for years in different climates and parts of the world. For this he urges as a fufficient reafon, the cold which is exceffively piercing, efpecially at the time of the year for curing the fifh. Sharp drying north winds reigning at this juncture, fetch out all the moifture, which is the internal caufe of corruption; befides at this time of curing no flies exift, and the few that appear about the latter end of the feafon, are kept off by the ftrong fmell of the fifh. Thus no flies come near them to lay their eggs, confequently no magots or worms grow in them, which is the external caufe of putrefaction.

is

is only laid to dry, and turned now and then by the women, and receives no damage from a little rain ; whereas the klip-fifh, after lying at firft three days in pickle, muft be wafhed in fea-water, then picked and laid out to dry, like the other fifh, and towards the evening made up in heaps, preffed with heavy ftones, and covered from the air. Every morning it muft be laid out again on the ftones to dry, and if it happens to rain in the day, it muft be immediately got under cover, becaufe the rain will quite fpoil it.

C H A P. LVII.

Concerning the ling.

THE ling is a fpecies of cod, but longer and narrower, from whence it takes the name of lange or ling. The inhabitants cure it in the manner they do cod, and make klip-fifh and flat-fifh of it, as may appear from the printed tax of prices of fifh. By law double the price is allowed for ling, and the merchants muft fo pay for it, which proves that it ought to be the beft. No great quantities are catched, but of fuch as are, they make klip-fifh as well as of cod, and that in perfection ; fo that this fifh is not peculiarly better in any other country *. This fort of fifh, or rather the way of curing the cod or ling, derives its name from the ftones taken off the cliffs when they lie upon the fifh to prefs them ; for klip fignifies a cliff, and fome authors derive the name of klip-fifh, or cliff-fifh, from being laid out upon the cliffs to dry.

* Mr. Anderfon fays, that the klip-fifh which the Icelanders make of ling, is not fo good as that of cod, for which reafon it is only ufed by the natives for their own confumption. He fays alfo that they are not very fuccefsful in their klip-fifh, which for the better part is indifferent, fpoils very foon, and therefore is not exported. To this he adds, that the different ways of curing fifh are peculiar to different countries, and he gives Norway the preference for round-fifh, Hitland for klip-fifh, and Iceland for dried fifh.

CHAP. LVIII.

Concerning the haddock.

THE haddock is called in the Iceland language ife, and is not one of the moſt contemptible fiſh about the iſland *. There is a great plenty of them, and at certain feaſons nothing elfe is caught. When they are fat, they are a well tafted fiſh. I know many at Copenhagen who prefer them to cod, but the reaſon is perhaps, becauſe they there are ſcarcer. The Daniſh merchants and the Icelanders make klip-fiſh of them, and I muſt confeſs, when cured in that manner, they are as good as cod. The merchants will not buy them of the Icelanders either cured this way or dried, but they buy them freſh, computing three haddocks worth two cods, which is a ſign that klip-fiſh is made of them, and that they are not much leſs than the cod †. Generally ſpeaking, they are as large as moſt of the cod. A vaſt many of them are dried, and when the company's ſhips are gone, I am certain, much more dried haddock remain in the iſland than cod ; becauſe the latter are uſually bought up by the merchants, in a far greater proportion than the former. The inhabitants among themſelves eſteem haddock equal to cod, and commonly mix and fell them together. The haddock is diſtinguiſhed by its ſcales, which are generally ſcraped off when klip-fiſh is intended to be made of it. It is alfo well known by two remarkable thick bones on the top of the head.

CHAP. LIX.

Concerning the whiting.

THE whiting, called in the Iceland language life, is here larger and fatter than I any where obſerved it. The fleſh is very delicate, and more like that of the haddock than the cod, becauſe white; and from thence deriving its name.

* Mr. Anderſon fays, that ſkiel-fiſh or ife, the fame as the haddock, is a ſpecies of cod. When boiled it flakes off from the bone in pretty thick, round flakes, and has remarkable ſcales, by which it is diſtinguiſhed from the reſt of the ſpecies.
† He alfo fays, that this fiſh is not fit to dry.

Y   Not

Not many being caught, they are mostly eaten fresh, and thus but few are dried, not being easily so preserved, and therefore not so fit for market.

CHAP. LX.

Concerning the sort of cod which the Icelanders call tisling.

THIS fish is called by the Icelanders tisling, which signifies a diminutive cod *. It is called by the Danes titling, and by that name is very well known at Copenhagen, to signify a small cod, and therefore nothing different from the young cod, as I before observed. There is a middle sort between this and the large, which they call stutting, and in Denmark, middle cod; but in the main, it is one and the same fish, and only different in size. This fish is variegated with grey, gold and black spots. In the summer it is lighter coloured than in winter, and those that have lain sometime near the shore in the weeds, have a brighter gold colour under the belly than the rest. The Icelanders generally make flat-fish of them, and when they deliver to the merchants great stacks of them, have as good a price as for the other dried fish †. They are also almost as common.

CHAP. LXI.

Concerning the cole-fish.

THE cole-fish, called by the Icelanders ypre, is, I believe, a species of cod, which it resembles, and is almost as large. It is a well tasted fish, and eaten by the Icelanders. When dried it is well known to be very good, though not quite equal to cod ‡. No large quantities being taken, not much is dried for use.

---

* Mr. Anderson says the tisling has small scales, which are hardly felt or discerned in the eating of it when boiled.

† The same Author says, that the Danish merchants make flat-fish of this small cod, and call them titlinger. They are in his opinion, a very delicate fish, and only made use of for presents to people of rank and fortune at Copenhagen, and consequently are seldom sent any where else.

‡ He also says the cole-fish is very lean, and such indifferent eating, that the Icelanders do not use it, unless in a scarcity of better.

CHAP.

C H A P. LXII.

Concerning flounders.

THE flounders here are very fat and fine, and are fit to dry, to be laid up for winter provision. This I have experienced myself, and have likewife feen them exported in fhips, whofe crew on throwing out five or fix nets, have catched great quantities, which they falted, dried, and carried away with them *. The inhabitants in general eat them frefh, falt being too precious. They never catch them otherwife than when they throw out their line for cod, and if then a flounder fhould bite, they catch it againft their will. It is true, in a few places they fifh for them with a net, and get vaft quantities, but all are for prefent ufe. To dry them, they muft be firft falted, and for want of falt, they cannot proceed to this operation.

C H A P. LXIII.

Concerning the turbot.

A GREAT many very large turbot are caught about Ice-land, fome fix foot long, and broad in proportion †. The inhabitants prepare a difh of them, which they call Riklingur, confifting of long flices cut lengthways, firft dried, and after-wards dreffed.

C H A P. LXIV.

Concerning mackarel.

MACKAREL is a fifh quite unknown to the Icelanders, either by that or any other name. As they come from the north, and take their peregrination through the ocean, and pafs by Hetland, Scotland, England, and ftill farther fouth, it

* Mr. Anderfon fays, the flounders are fo very fat, that when dried, they will not keep, but prefently turn red near the bones, therefore as fpoiled, they are not fit for exportation.

† The fame Author fays, that fome turbot taken on the coaft of Iceland, have weighed 400 lb.

is

is poffible they may mix with other fifh about Iceland, though they never ftay, or ever are caught fo as to be known: this feveral of the natives have affured me. They catch a fifh here in feveral places, chiefly weftward, which they call fteenbidder. It is not the fame with that of this name in Denmark. In fize it is nearly as large as a cod, of a dark colour, no fcales, fhort head, fmall mouth, with a great many fharp teeth, and in afpect very fierce. The fifhermen take a great deal of care when they catch this fifh, that it does them no mifchief. It is without doubt the *lupus marinus*, and may be called the fea-pike, as refembling very much the frefh water pike. Its flefh very good is eaten both frefh and dried by the Icelanders. At certain feafons this fifh is more frequently caught than at others, and in general is of great ufe and benefit to the inhabitants. There is another fifh much like this, and called by the Icelanders Klir, which is very good eating, and is caught in feveral places, but not in fuch abundance. Rödmaven, or red-belly is a fifh I before mentioned, in difcourfing of the fea-gull, and therefore will not repeat what I faid. It is caught in great abundance with hooks, nets, and with fpears, much after the manner of the eel-fpear. It affords a delicate difh, being dreffed feveral ways, and is very good when falted a little, dried, and then fmoaked. Of the fame form and fhape as the rödmaven, is a fifh frequently caught, which the Icelanders call graae-maven, or grey-belly. It is fomewhat larger, and very good eating. Both are reckoned to be the fame fpecies, the rödmave being called the male, and the graaemave the female; becaufe in the former they never find a hard-row, nor in the latter a foft. The thornback, which the Icelanders call fkata, is in great plenty, and is a very fine fifh, efpecially when cured in the manner of klip-fifh. The taxprice demonftrates it to be a good and defirable fifh, being rated at double the price of a large cod. Karve is a well tafted fifh, and is fometimes caught with the hook, but not in any plenty. By fhape and tafte it feems to me to be the perch. Thefe are the principal fifh of the fmaller kind about the coaft, which are of great ufe and benefit to the inhabitants; I fhall now give an account of the larger fort in the ocean.

2   C H A P.

C H A P. LXV.

Concerning the whale.

WHALES of all kinds are in abundance about Iceland. They have particular names, and to enumerate them all would make a treatife. The great Greenland whale often appears on this coaft, and becaufe he has a fmooth back without fins, the Icelanders call him fletbakar, that is, fmooth-back *. The fand whale is of a quite different kind. Several other forts of large whales appear about the coaft, and in the creeks and large bays, as in Hvalfiorden, which from thence derives its name, and in many more on the weft coaft. I have feen ten or twelve at a time in Hvalfiorden, which ftopped up the entrance. They generally arrive there about the latter end of July, or beginning of Auguft, and are not a fmall fort, the Icelanders having catched fome 200 and 240 feet long †. In order to catch them, a boat goes out and endeavours to get as near the fifh as poffible. An expert perfon being at hand to ftrike him with an iron harpoon, as foon as the blow is given, the boat immediately makes off as quick as poffible. The harpoon is ftamped with the mark of him that ftruck it in the fifh. The whale not being able to furvive the wound, if hit well, dies, and floats to fome part of the coaft; but if the wind fets from

---

* Mr. Anderfon fays, the great Greenland whale, not caring to venture clofe to Iceland, for fear of fhallows, keeps out in the fathomlefs ocean about Spitfberg, and under the north pole.

† The fame Author fays, that as foon the Icelanders obferve the whale in purfuit of the herrings towards the coaft, they without delay get into their boats, and taking their harpoons, fpears and knives with them, row away, and endeavour to get behind him, and as clofe to his body as poffible. When the wind fets to the fhore they throw into the fea a quantity of all forts of blood, which they provide themfelves with on purpofe. The wind blowing it about the flying fifh, they row gently after, and the fifh perceiving himfelf purfued, is for turning about, but finding the fea all bloody, which he detefts, and rather than fwim back through it, he turns again, and driving towards the fhore, runs a-ground, or into narrow creeks, where he is catched. The wind happening to be unfavourable, they have recourfe to another method, and this is, by throwing large ftones into the fea at the whale, and fetting up a hideous noife to frighten him; whereupon finding himfelf purfued, he darts off with precipitation, runs a-ground, and cannot ftir. So foon as they have frightened him a-ground, they all furround and give him ftab upon ftab, till by the violent effufion of blood he expires. Then they cut off all the blubber they can, and as they are not very dainty; take fome of the flefh alfo, and carry it home.

the

the fhore, is fometimes carried out to fea and loft. If the fifh comes afhore, by the laws of Iceland, a certain fhare belongs to him that owns the harpoon, and the proprietor of the land where he ftops has the reft. This is all the art they make ufe of to catch whales, and is the full extent of their ingenuity. But as they are now provided with fifhing tackle, harpoons, and other implements, and a perfon that underftands the bufinefs to teach them, I prefume whales will not for the future eafily efcape them *. The fins are fold to the Danifh merchants, and are not fmall, as may be concluded from the above-mentioned fizes of the whales. The blubber of the whale they melt down in large pots, in which they firft have put fome water. The train that fwims on the top they continue the fkimming off as long as there is any †. The flefh that remains in the pot has no trainy tafte in their opinion. They take and put it in their fyre, which is as four as vinegar, and when macerated for fome time in this liquor, it becomes very good eating. This is the way many of the Icelanders prepare this flefh for ufe. I have been told by thofe who have eat of it, that it is very good; but it will not be amifs to obferve, that as the flefh of all whales is not fit for eating, the following general rule to know which is, may be eafily attended to. The flefh of thofe whales that have teeth are not fit to eat; but thofe without teeth may be proper food.

C H A P. LXVI.

Concerning the porpus.

THE porpus, which the Icelander calls nife, is from five to eight foot long. They roll themfelves about in the fea, and move but flowly. Their flefh is very good. The Icelanders kill a great many with their harpoons. Sometimes they

* Mr. Anderfon fays, that the fins being but fmall, the Danifh merchants do not much regard them, and that the Icelanders have fuch miferable tools, that they cannot cut them off; for which reafon they are left on. They are fhaped like a fabreblade, are of a horny fubftance, and adhere on each fide of the upper jaw-bone, in a hanging manner. This is what is commonly called whale-bone. Its ufes are various.

† The fame Author fays, they throw the fat into a veffel or hogfhead, and letting it lie a quarter of a year, it melts by degrees, and leaks through; that which leaks through in that time, is the fineft and beft, and muft not be poured off, or boiled up.

chafe

chafe them afhore, being eafily frightened, and they kill them
in June as well as in other months. None here fuppofe them to
be blinder at one time of the year than another. They fwim
not quicker, but that two men in a boat may keep up with,
manage and take them, and this both before and after the month
of June; for their fight is the fame all the year round. There
is a whale called the fpring-whale, and very often eighteen foot
long, which will jump furprifingly in the water, and take great
delight in purfuing boats; but when they jump out of the
water to throw themfelves on a boat, their eyelids fall over their
eyes and blind them *.

C H A P. LVII.

Concerning the fea-calf †.

THE fea-calf is called by the Icelanders haakal. They
catch a great many by a fort of machine which they
fink to the bottom of the ocean, with a buoy faftened to it, that
floats on the furface. The hooks are rivetted to iron chains to
prevent their biting them off. When the people go out to fee
what fuccefs they have had with their machine, they find fometimes twelve or fixteen faft to the hooks, which by tying the
chains to the boat-ftern they drag afhore. This turns out a
very profitable fifhery. Though the flefh of this fifh is good
eating, it has notwithftanding been obferved, that thofe that
have eat much of it frefh, or often, were afflicted with fevere fits
of illnefs, or died fuddenly. It is therefore now not eaten, till
it has hung up for a twelvemonth, and all the fat is melted away ;
then it taftes like fmoaked or dried falmon. Once at an entertainment, a Danifh merchant eat of it, and believed it fuch, till
he was undeceived. No train is extracted from the flefh of this
fifh, but the liver is fo large, that it often yields thirty gallons of

---

* Mr. Anderfon fays, the porpus is a fpecies of whale from five to eight foot long.
They fwim fo very faft, and are fo quick in the water, that they are with difficulty
got at. The Icelanders would be unfuccefsful in their queft after them, were it not
for the extraordinary circumftance of their becoming blind in the month of June.
Our author fays that Mr. Anderfon confounds the fpring-whale with the porpus.
† Martin in his defcription of the weft ifles of Scotland, calls this fifh the white
fhark.

very

very fine oil. In sea-calves eighteen foot long, livers have been found of so prodigious a size, as frequently to produce the quantity of two thirty-six gallon casks of oil.

C H A P. LXVIII.

Concerning the sword-fish or saw-fish.

THERE are sword-fish, or saw-fish, as well as other large fish about Iceland; but as nothing peculiar is observable in them, I will omit further speaking of them *.

C H A P. LXIX.

Concerning sea-bulls, and sea-cows.

IT is commonly reported, that the noise and bellowing of these animals make the cows ashore run mad; but none here ever saw any of these supposed animals, or noticed the bad effects of their bellowing.

C H A P. LXX.

Concerning the seal.

A VAST many seals are seen about this island, which the inhabitants distinguish by the names of land-seals, island-seals, and Greenland seals. The first the smallest, and most common, are always near the land, and run up the creeks and rivers to hunt the salmon, salmon-trout, trout, and such nice fish. Island-seals are the largest, and so called, because they harbour in the little islands about the coast, and prefer those that are uninhabited and desolate, in order to be quiet and at rest. The Greenland are as large as the island-seals, but yet are thought to be of a different species. They arrive annually in the month of December, especially about the northern parts of the country, and generally stay till May, at which time those that escape

---

* Mr. Anderson says, that the saw-fish is so eager in pursuit of the seals, that they will often jump ashore to escape them, and that he has been told, that the sea-bull's head is like that of an ox, and body and legs like those of a seal, and that their bellowing makes the land cows mad, or to run staring after the sound.

the Icelanders depart. They come in great numbers, and are caught in nets in some of the bays and creeks where they harbour. Twenty or thirty nets, each full twenty fathom long, are so ranged like a wilderness or decoy, that they cannot well escape, but must be caught in some of them. When the people draw their nets, they sometimes find two hundred of them, and seldom under sixty, each of which they value at two rixdollars, they yield a deal of train-oil, and their skins are very fine. In the district of Oefiord, the inhabitants seldom use nets, but kill them with a harpoon, at which they are very dextrous, and get a great many. They can take their aim at forty or fifty yards distance, and throw a harpoon fastened to a line, and hit their mark. The Greenland seals are ten foot long, and few under four. I don't find that they appear in any other part of the island, perhaps they may be westward; but what I have related is certainly true. The island seals are caught in abundance about the uninhabited islands, where they think themselves secure. Several men go together for this purpose to these islands, where they watch them when they come ashore to bask themselves in the sun. As soon as they perceive them laid out, they fall upon them with clubs, and knock them down, often to the amount of a hundred at a time. In the same manner they kill the land seals, which are not near so plenty as the Greenland, though met with all round the island. Such as are taken southward are generally shot with a gun that carries a great way. This is an article that ought not to be omitted in a genuine description of this island, the seals that are caught about it, being of great benefit and advantage to the inhabitants.

C H A P. LXXI.

Concerning fresh water fish.

I SHOULD be tedious, were I to enumerate the many rivers that abound with salmon in this island. In the northern Oefiord, Skagefiord, Hunnevatns, Borgefiord, Guldbringe, and Arnes districts, vast quantities of salmon are taken, as also in other places, but not in such abundance. It is a general remark, that where rivers run from the fresh water lakes in the

A a   country

country frequented by trout, there falmon ufually go up from the fea *. It is well known, that the falmon always go againft the ftream, and againft any water-fall, and will jump to an incredible height over the falling current. Their way of catching falmon, is by a kind of machine, which they call falmon-chefts, with covers, locks and keys. Thefe are put in the middle of each arm of the rivers that run to the fea. The river is ftopped up on each fide of the cheft, to prevent the falmon getting by, and on the fide of the cheft that turns to the fea, there is an aperture big enough for the largeft falmon to pafs through. Pieces of hoops are nailed clofe to each other on the infide, and about the edges of the aperture. They are fharp-pointed within the cheft, and are made pliable, that the falmon may eafily bend them open, to make their way in. By their elafticity, they fpring together again when the falmon enter, and it is impoffible for them to get back, the points of the hoops turning againft them, and keeping them confined, till thofe that are on the watch come and open the cover, and take them out alive †. In the river Heller, and in other fmall rivers, they ufe nets for catching them, which they do in great plenty, by reafon of the fhoals of them that are met with in various parts of the ifland. Befides falmon, are vaft quantities of trout, and of three or four different forts in the lakes of Myvatne and Tingvalle, which are thirty or forty miles in circumference. Of this delicate fifh they have fuch abundance, efpecially in Myvatne, that they dry and make flat-fifh of them. They are exceeding good this way. Some falt them, and in fome places there is fuch plenty, that the people live upon them all the year round, dreffing and making them palatable feveral different ways. I have eat very fine eels here, but the Icelanders in general, having an averfion to them, never trouble themfelves about them. It is not therefore known whether there be any great quantity. I do not think there are

---

* Mr. Anderfon fays, that near Holm in Ellera by Kleppee, as well as in other deep rivers, and where the water falls from the rocks, there are always falmon. Our author calls this river Heller, and fays it may be always forded, and that there is no ftrong current or water-fall in it.

† He alfo fays, they catch falmon in what they call chefts, which are laid a-crofs the rivers. Thefe chefts are made of lathes nailed together, through which the falmon can make fhift to pafs, but cannot return.

other

other forts of frefh water fifh in Iceland; but as thefe are the niceft and moft delicate we have in Denmark, I thought them worth notice, and of great confequence to Iceland.

CHAP. LXXII.

Concerning fnakes.

NO fnakes of any kind are to be met with throughout the whole ifland *.

CHAP. LXXIII.

Concerning infects and vermin.

NO country on the globe is lefs troubled with infects and fuch fort of vermin. Spiders there are a few, but beetles and horfe-flies are fcarce known. The only troublefome thing of the kind are gnats, which are pretty large, and in great numbers in the northern diftrict, and coldeft part of the country, efpecially about the lake Myvatne, which from thence derives its name †. They torment the people as well as the cattle, and travellers are obliged to hang a piece of gauze over their face to keep them off; for their fting fmarts to a great degree. This proves that the cold is not too fevere for fuch fmall infects to breed and live in. The northern diftrict abounding more in wood, gnats are more frequent there, chiefly by the fide of rivers where bufhes grow. I before obferved, that where fifh is cured, a great many flies will gather about them, when they lie out to dry. No other forts of infects are met with. When much dry weather has happened, and it afterwards rains, worms will appear in abundance, crawling about the ground, as in other countries. Another fort of worm appears in very rainy weather, which as the inhabitants imagine, falls with the rain ‡. It is

* Mr. Anderfon fays, it is owing to the exceffive cold that no fnakes are found in Iceland.

† The fame Author fays, that this country breeds but few infects on account of the long and exceffive cold, and for want of trees and bufhes; fuch as it does, are chiefly horfe-flies, which he tells us lay their eggs in the noftrils, and the innermoft edge of the *Foramen ani* of cattle, where they are hatched by the natural heat of the animal.

‡ He alfo fays, that when it rains, fo many rain-worms, *Lumbrici Terreftres*, appear, that people think they come down with the rain.

green,

green, and in shape and size like a silk-worm. When about half grown, they hurt the grass very much wherever they fall. However, they are not common, and it is but a little spot of ground they occupy.

C H A P. LXXIV.

Concerning mice.

THERE are a great many mice in this island; for as all are obliged to lay up a stock of provision in their houses, the mice find sufficient store. The merchants, who leave the factories in the winter, lock up their houses during that time, and at their return in the spring, find by their provisions, that they have had many guests, their tubs of flour being partly emptied, and their dried fish gnawed and eaten by them. Undoubtedly, they can endure the cold; for no fire is kept all the time in these houses *.

C H A P. LXXV.

Concerning the sun when above and below the horizon.

IN the northern part of the island, taking in the divisions of Hunnevatns, Skagefiord, and Oefiord, the sun is not seen constantly above the horizon at any time. This is only perceived

* Mr. Anderson says, very few mice can live in Iceland, upon account of the piercing cold and scarcity of nourishment in the ground, where they presently dig into sulphur, or come against a rock. He relates a story told him by a person who averred that he had several times made the experiment, and found it matter of fact. This was in the church-yard of the ancient cloyster or abbey of Widöe, which has this peculiar property, that as soon as a mouse is let go upon the ground, it instantly expires. His opinion in the case is, that the sulphureous vapours, by exhaling stronger here than any where else, must be the chief cause of the death of the animal, and so much the more, as the ground all over the island is nothing but sulphur, with a lay of mould over it, and this church-yard impregnated perhaps therewith in a stronger degree than any where else, which may easily be discovered on the spot, either with a candle, if not too dangerous, or by digging in the ground and smelling to it. Our author turns this story into ridicule, and assures us, there is no sulphur in the ground at Widöe; but that it is one of the finest and most fertile islands about Iceland, and that if there was sulphur, it could not possibly bear such fine grass as it does. He says, that by smelling to the ground, he could not discover the least odour of sulphur in it. Besides, it was formerly the residence of some dainty monks, who, as experienced in the art of indulging themselves, would have made choice of a wholsomer and more pleasant spot to reside in, if this did not serve their purpose.

in

in the extreme northern points at cape de Nord, and at Langenefs, where the fun is feen, fome time before the fummer folftice, and fome time after, perpetually above the horizon, and
in appearance about the height of a man *. In the fouth part
of the ifland we reckon the fun's altitude at the winter folftice,
about two degrees above the horizon, including refraction. I
was not at the northern part of the ifland, but fome learned and
ingenious men, who lived there many years, informed me, that
in the fhorteft day in winter, they fee the fun one hour above
the horizon, and have four hours day-light, befides twilight.
This is the actual cafe to the northward; but not in the moft
extreme northern points. In the divifions of Strand and Ife-
fiords, the days are fhorter, but not fo fhort as to be deftitute of
refractionis beneficio. An hour and a half, or three quarters twilight, continue during two entire months; but no fuch place is
known fouthward, the fun at the winters folftice being feen three
hours above the horizon, and the days full fix hours long; for
crepufculum matutinum & vefpertinum, or the break of day in
the morning, and twilight in the evening, continue much longer
in Iceland than in Denmark; becaufe the fun is a great while
before it rifes and fets, going a long way, as it were, clofe under the horizon before it entirely difappears, that is, the circle it
defcribes under the horizon, being more oblique than in Denmark, or more fouthern parts, where it rifes and fets more per-
pendicularly, and therefore makes the *crepufculum* of a fhorter
duration †. Confequently, the fun's drawing near to the horizon,

* Mr. Anderfon fays, that on the north fide of the ifland from the middle of June,
to the latter end of July, the fun is perpetually above the horizon, and to appearance
the outer ring is upwards of a man's height from the furface of the fea above the
horizon.

Our author argues againft this affertion, and fays, that even illiterate people know
that the fun's altitude is the fame at an equal diftance from the tropic on either fide;
and as the fun enters the tropic the 21ft of June, there are at moft but fix days from
the middle of that month; but from the time the fun enters the tropic to the latter
end of July are forty-one days, confequently there muft be a great miftake in this
account.

† Mr. Anderfon fays, that in December and January, the fun is entirely invifible,
except on the high rocks that turn to the fun, where a little light may appear, and this
undoubtedly only in confequence of *refractionis beneficii,* or a twilight of one hour and
a half; or three quarters. Our author obferves, that here is a like miftake in regard
to the time of the fun's being invifible, as was before about the time of his being
conftantly above the horizon. The fun cannot be fo many days invifible under the

B b

horizon,

zon, and leaving it much quicker than where the circle is more oblique, muſt be the reaſon why the days or day-light in Iceland, is much longer in proportion to the time of the ſun's being above the horizon than in more ſouthern parts. Although I knew it to be ſo, I could not imagine it had ſo great an effect as I experienced, being ſurpriſed to find the days almoſt as long here at the winter ſolſtice as in Copenhagen, though the ſun was not ſo long above the horizon. Hence it may alſo be accounted for, why the days increaſe faſter in Iceland, and particularly after the days and nights are equal. In the beginning of May, hardly any night paſſes but one may travel and do buſineſs as in the day-time, and in the middle of May, one may ſee to read all night, and that even in the ſouth part of the iſland. Northward it begins ſooner, and is much lighter.

C H A P. LXXVI.

Concerning the aurora borealis, *or north light.*

THE north light appears in every reſpect, after the ſame manner it does in Denmark, except that it is more frequent, and happens without any rule or order, not depending of the days lengthening or ſhortening *. Neither does it appear juſt upon the ſun's ſetting; for I have often not obſerved it till eight, nine or ten o'clock at night. Sometimes it has laſted only an hour, ſometimes longer, and ſometimes it has appeared by intervals all night; but not always ſo. It appears as bright as in Denmark, and is very ſerviceable to travellers, but not ſufficient light to do any labour or work by †. Nothing invariable is ob-

horizon as he is viſibly above; for the refraction makes the ſun appear longer above the horizon in the ſummer than he actually is, and *vice verſa* to appear fewer days under the horizon in winter than he ought. Notwithſtanding Mr. Anderſon makes the ſun remain half a month longer below the horizon in winter than above it in ſummer, which is quite againſt the nature of the thing; for there may be places where the ſun is above the horizon eight days conſtantly at the ſummer ſolſtice, but never quite inviſible at the winter ſolſtice, and both from the refraction which we know is very ſtrong at the horizon.

* Mr. Anderſon ſays, as the days decreaſe in Iceland, the north light begins to appear, and encreaſes in duration and brightneſs as the days decreaſe, lightening all night long in the winter, and gradually diſappearing as the days begin to increaſe.

† The ſame Author ſays, when the ſky is clear of ſnow, rain, and clouds, or when a bright ſtar-light ſky appears, the ſun being ſet, and only twilight, then the north light is ſeen, which laſts all night, flaſhing and dancing ſo bright, that it does not only reſemble the light and brightneſs of a full moon, but even ſurpaſſes it.

ſervable

fervable in the fhooting forth of its rays. I have as often feen it fhoot forth from the fouth as from the north, and it often appears in a bright broad bow from eaft to weft, and will remain fo a good while. Sometimes it plays all over the fky, fhooting all its rays to the zenith, and feldom fixes in clear and diftinct bows to the fouth and north, as it frequently does in Denmark *. The Icelanders have no notion of its foretelling what weather will happen, farther, than if coloured and playing about, they then think it will be windy; if ftill and bright, they expect fine weather; and if the bow remains the whole evening in the fouth, and afterwards in the north, they imagine either rain or fnow will fall; but thefe conjectures are liable to great miftakes, neither do they depend upon them. I cannot fay, that the Icelanders think the north lights more frequent now than formerly, though it is thought fo in Denmark †. The learned Mayran has publifhed an excellent treatife on the *aurora borealis,* or north light.

CHAP. LXXVII.

Concerning thunder and meteors.

IT thunders very feldom in Iceland. In the north thunder fometimes happens in fummer; but in the other parts of the ifland, not till about Michaelmas, and very rarely in winter. During the whole time I continued in Iceland, I heard it thunder but once, and this only three or four claps about noon, in the middle of June. I allow it may have thundered in other parts of the ifland that year; for Iceland is fo large, that the thunder cannot be heard every where; fo that upon the whole,

---

* Mr. Anderfon fays, the north light always fhoots from the north or north-weft, to the fouth, and fometimes fills the whole fky.

† He alfo afferts, that as far as he can fee, it is plain and demonftrable, the north light can have no other origin than the ftrong fulphureous vapours, which readily take fire, and muft be very high in the air, becaufe feen at fuch a great diftance. In warm climates, fuch vapours take fire and vanifh in lightening before they get to any great height; but here near the north pole, on account of the great coldnefs of the earth, they afcend to the uppermoft part of the atmofphere, where being collected, condenfed, and compreffed, at laft by frequent collifions take fire, and then like a fine piece of fire-work, dart their rays about. Our author fays, that the learned Mayran does not derive the caufe from the bowels of the earth, but traces it much higher.

it

it is plain, that not much thunder happens in this ifland, and that when it does, it is neither peculiar to fummer nor winter *. The thunder at Copenhagen is by far ftronger, as I am credibly informed by thofe that have heard it feveral times in both places. *Ignis fatuus*, *ignes lambentes*, and fuch like meteors, are feldom feen in Iceland, the air being in general too clear for collecting them †. It is true, I have feen ftars fhoot, but not fo frequently as at Copenhagen.

CHAP. LXXVIII.

Concerning parhelions, or mock funs.

I NEVER faw but two parhelions in Iceland, both which happened in the month of April, and were fucceeded by fine weather ‡. The firft was in April 1750, at which time two coloured funs appeared about the fun, and were attended with mild thawing weather. The fecond I obferved in April 1751. Both were bright in the forenoon, and one having paffed before the fun in the ring, vanifhed in the afternoon. The other was afterwards feen only behind the fun. This parhelion was fucceeded by fine mild and calm weather, as it had been before for fome time. I never faw any other in Iceland. I have been told by fome, that they appear but feldom, and when they do, it is moft commonly in the fpring of the year, and the people as well as in Denmark, think they bode bad weather which does not always follow more in one place than in the other.

---

* Mr. Anderfon affigns the fame reafon for there being but little thunder in Iceland in the fummer, as he does for the *aurora borealis*; but adds, that it is by far more violent in winter.

 † The fame author fays when it fnows, there appears in particular a number of *ignes lambentes*, &c. Undoubtedly in a country where they deal fo much in train and fifh, there cannot want matter to produce thefe appearances. Such flames and lights as they appear to be in the dark, adhere to all their clubs and fticks, mafts, fails, and oars, hats and caps, or any thing elfe. The poor people, fimple and ftupid as in moft countries, are frightened by this fire, though they cannot light any thing by it, or ever faw an inftance of the kind. As foon as they take notice of it, they run into their houfes, fhut the doors, and are forely afraid left it fhould get to their hearths, and incorporate with the other fire, and fo fet the whole building in flames.

 ‡ He alfo fays, that about the latter end of fummer, parhelions often appear, which are fucceeded by ftormy and bad weather, as the people ufually prognofticate.

2

CHAP.

CHAP. LXXIX.

Concerning the seasons of the year.

THE meteorological tables hereto annexed, plainly shew when the seasons change, and from them it may appear, that in the year 1750 and 1751, the spring-season was very favourable *. Grass with other plants began to shoot both these years in the middle of April. The autumn was also very favourable, and as fine and as mild as ever I saw in Denmark, which I was very much surprised at. The same happened in 1749. The first nights frost was then not till the 29th of October. The day following there was some snow, which only fell that day, the weather afterwards becoming for some time rainy. In 1750, the 9th of October, was the first of frost and snow in the night; but the same ceased in a few days, and the weather was very mild again for a considerable time. In regard to the spring, my observations shew, that on the 15th of April 1750, it began to be clear and calm, and fine spring weather ensued, just as in Denmark. In 1751, it began about the middle of April, and continued fine and mild, the grass springing up in many places the beginning of the month; and indeed, finer weather could not be wished for. The thermometer all the year round will confirm how good the seasons are, which I could not have imagined, had I not known it by experience. My observations will also sufficiently demonstrate, that the transition from summer to winter is not so sudden, but that there is an intervening spring and autumn. The Icelanders reckon their summer from the Thursday that falls between the 18th and 24th of April, and their winter from the Friday between the 18th and 24th of October. They may compute so; but nature will not hold to that standard; heat and cold scarce ever admitting so sudden a transition; and thus it is their spring and autumn must happen when the days and nights are equal, which time they themselves often call by the name of spring and autumn. Though the Ice-

---

* Mr. Anderson says, the Icelanders have but the two seasons of summer and winter, which suddenly change from one to the other, without any intermediate milder weather, as spring or autumn.

landers

landers reckon their feafons in this manner, which makes fummer and winter, except one day, of equal length; yet it muft
be allowed, that the winter is much longer. It is fo even in
Denmark, and of confequence fhould be of greater continuance
here. It fnows and hails fometimes in the fummer, which it
equally does in Denmark. How great the heat is in fummer,
may be determined by the meteorological obfervations. It is
certainly very warm fometimes in the fummer, but I cannot fay
that it ever is fo fultry, that there is a neceffity of throwing off
all cloaths. When the days were hot, I found the nights fo in
proportion, which at that time cannot be very cold, the fun being but three hours below the horizon *. A little fnow or hail
may happen to fall in the fummer, but it does not come of a
fudden, and may be perceived fome days before, by the coldnefs of the air, which is alfo obfervable in Norway and Denmark. A like quantity of fnow does not fall every year, fome
years being very fnowy, and others not: neither does it fnow
all over the ifland with one and the fame wind, each place having a particular wind that brings fnow and rain †. The two
winters I was there, efpecially the laft, but little fnow fell in the
fouth part of the ifland, and not fo much as commonly at Copenhagen. It hardly fnowed above two days together, and in
frofty weather perhaps not for a fortnight or three weeks. When
it thaws, the fnow is prefently gone, and the cattle are turned
out to feed, and even find fome nourifhment on the ground,
during the whole winter. In the north the fnow is in much
greater abundance, and fometimes falls very thick and heavy,
burying the houfes, efpecially where they are fituated among
rocks, (from which the fnow tumbles down) and making all the
lower parts level. Though this fometimes happens in fome few
places, it cannot from thence be inferred, that the whole ifland
is in this condition, it being evident, that to the fouthward, and

---

* Mr. Anderfon fays, it is fo hot in the day time in fummer, that the people are
obliged to throw off all their cloaths; and in the night fo exceffively cold, that they
cannot cover themfelves fufficiently; and in the morning, he adds, all the country
round is feen covered with fnow.

† The fame Author fays, that vaft quantities of fnow fall in the winter; that it
fnows moft commouly with eafterly winds, and that the houfes and fields, &c. are
all covered with heaps of fnow.

other

other parts, the like feldom, or ever happens. In the north, a
north wind generally brings fnow along with it, as does alfo the
Ice that comes floating from Greenland, which befides occafions
a fharp nipping cold, and often very fenfibly felt in the fouth.
As the north wind brings fnow to the northward, fo in the fame
manner other parts of the ifland have their particular winds,
which blow from the fea. Hence it cannot be properly faid,
that fuch a wind occafions fuch weather all over the ifland; becaufe every part of this great ifland having fomething peculiar to
it, it is not fo eafy to give a genuine and faithful defcription,
which requires a very ftrict enquiry, and thorough examination.
In the months of February and March, very fevere weather fometimes happens, and often to the north in April *. But generally fpeaking, the month of April is very mild, and though
the preceding were very fevere, which may be feen in the meteorological obfervations, fharp frofts having exifted from time to
time in the winter months of 1751, that is, in January, February, and March, yet April was very mild and fine. It may
alfo be feen, that in the year 1750 and 1751, fouth and eaft
winds blew chiefly in April, but very little north wind, efpecially the laft year; and what is moft to be wondered at is,
that of the few north winds that blew, fcarce any were attended
with frofts, except in the night time, and thefe but inconfider-
able.

C H A P. LXXX.

Concerning the weather.

MANY days, and fometimes weeks, pafs without any perceptible brifk gale of wind, the weather being quite
calm and ferene, as the meteorological tables may fhew †. The
wind is changeable here as in other countries, but not generally
fo high; though I will allow, that the weather is frequently

---

* Mr. A. lerfon fays he has been informed, that they have moft exceffive cold
weather, pa ticularly in April, as then north winds conftantly blow, and bring with
them more and more fenfibly piercing and cutting icy particles from the more remote
icy mountains under the north pole.

† He alfo fays, that the wind in this ifland is never fettled, but continually changing and veering about.

more

more ftormy than in Denmark, which is partly owing to the
fituation of the mountains.   It may be calm in one place, and
perhaps ten or twelve Englifh miles farther, exceeding tempeftuous *.   During my ftay in the ifland, two very great ftorms
happened.   When the weather is fine in fummer, the night is
frequently ufhered in with a land-wind all over the ifland, and
between nine and eleven in the forenoon, generally comes a fea
breeze, which lafts till five in the afternoon.   Thefe land-winds
and fea breezes, are in no refpect tempeftuous, neither are they
attended with heavy rains, or other inclemencies of the air.
During the land-winds, the weather fets generally fair ; but the
fea breezes often bring with them rain or fnow, according to the
time of the year.   Thus a fouth-eaft, or fouth-weft wind ufually brings rain or fnow to the fouthward, whilft to the northward
there is fine, clear, frofty, or dry weather ; and *vice verfa*, a
north wind caufes fnow or rain to the northward, whilft the
fouth parts enjoy fine dry weather.   At Beffefted fome high
winds have happened as well with north and north-eaft winds, as
with fouth-eaft.

CHAP. LXXXI.

Concerning the ebb and flood, or the tides.

THE ebbing and flowing of the tide, is the fame as in
other countries, that is, twice in twenty-four hours, and
changing every fix.   The tides are always higheft about the new
and full moon, and particularly when the days and nights are
of equal length.   The ebb and flood are called by the Icelanders
flod and *fiöre*.   It feems as if it were a rule in Iceland, that the
wind, rain, and fnow, fhould, each at times, increafe with the
flood in this manner, that if the wind rifes a little at ebb-tide,
it grows ftronger and ftronger with the flood ; and though it
may feem to be allayed when the tide is out, yet it generally rifes
again on the return of the flood, and gradually increafes as the
water fwells : but if it be ftill, when the tide is coming in, it

* Mr. Anderfon fays, that a north-weft wind brings fine weather, at leaft to the
fouthward, and on the contrary, a fouth-weft bad weather; but a fouth-eaft, very
great ftorms.

most

moſt commonly continues ſo. With regard to the height of the tide-water, I have obſerved, that at the higheſt ſpring tides it riſes to ſixteen feet, and at other times to about twelve.

CHAP. LXXXII.

Concerning the ſea water.

THE ſea-water round this iſland, at leaſt in ſome places, is much ſalter than in other countries, and there is good reaſon to think ſo, by its leaving in ſummer the rocks incruſtated with ſalt, when the tide is down, and the moiſture evaporated. The country people ſcrape it off with knives, and in holes in the cliffs at low water, find it ſometimes in great abundance. It appears by ancient deeds of donations in catholic times, to the clergy of eſtates and privileges, that among other things, the emoluments ariſing from ſalt-works were aſſigned them: even certain tracts of land, as Langeneſs and other places, deſtined for the ſame purpoſe, have been annexed to the biſhopric in the north, and ſtill belong to it. To this may be added, the experiments made to refine ſalt to greater advantage than in Denmark, which ſufficiently demonſtrates, that the ſea water here, contains more ſalt than is uſual in other places. It never freezes to ſuch a degree in Iceland, ſo as to cover the ſea about the ſhores with ice: the reaſon is, becauſe the ſea runs almoſt every where quite up to the land, which, together with a conſiderable ebb and flow, ſo keeps the water in agitation, that it cannot admit of being frozen, even by the moſt intenſe cold. It is true, notwithſtanding that in ſmall creeks and bays with a narrow entrance, the ſea water is often quite frozen up, chiefly upon account of its being ſheltered by the land from the boiſterous waves of the ocean. Hence it is, that greater quantities of ſea water are frozen in the ſouth than in the north; becauſe abounding more in creeks and bays; but it has not been known in the memory of man, that the ſea was ever covered with ice, ſo as to hinder the iſlanders from going out to fiſh. The only ice that incommodes them in the north, and hinders them from putting out to ſea, is that which comes floating from Greenland; ſometimes

D d ſpreading

spreading itſelf many miles about the north coaſt, and in appearance, like another country joined thereto, and ſometimes
filling the eye with the reſemblance of mountains and dales, with
live animals; flying and clambering up and down, as falcons,
bears, foxes, &c *. This ice occaſions exceſſive cold, and thick
fogs, in the northern parts, which alſo in ſome meaſure extend
to the ſouthern; for when a cold ſpring happens, the inhabitants immediately conclude, that great quantities of Greenland
ice lie to the northward; and hence it is, that thoſe who have
been only in thoſe parts, may imagine it is ſo all round the iſland.

C H A P. LXXXIII.

*Concerning the climate of Iceland, and the conſtitution of the
inhabitants.*

FROM my meteorological obſervations, and what I remarked relating to the weather, it is plain, that Iceland is
a healthy country to live in. I can partly avouch by my own
experience, that the air and weather of this country will agree
better with a ſtranger, than the air and weather in Denmark
would with an Icelander †. The ſummer's heat in Denmark
would be rather too much for him, though not much hotter there
than here; whereas the ſummer in Iceland would be quite agreeable to any foreigner, the air being neither thick nor ſultry, nor
the winters in general colder than in Denmark. The only ˛dif-
ference I find between Denmark and Iceland is, that in the
latter, ſtormy and windy weather is more frequent. But it cannot from thence be concluded that the country is unhealthy;
rather the reverſe ſhould take place, as by theſe winds and ſtorms
the air is purified, and rendered more wholeſome ‡. The Ice-

* Mr. Anderſon ſays, the ſea is ſalter than elſewhere about Iceland, which he at-
tributes to the exceſſive cold that freezes ſo much of the ſea-water without the ſalt
into vaſt flakes. The high winds by carrying away the better part of theſe flakes,
whatever is left behind muſt of conſequence abound with much ſalt; therefore the
ſea-water about Iceland may be deemed ſalter than in other countries.

† The ſame Author is of opinion, that Iceland is a healthy country for the natives,
and thoſe that from their early youth have been accuſtomed to the air and weather.

‡ He alſo ſays, they live to a great age, and many of them to a hundred and upwards, enjoying life chearful and undiſturbed, and being very little acquainted with
the weakneſſes and ailments that attend old age in other countries.

landers

landers are endowed with good bodily ftrength, by being inured to hard labour from their youth, but not from childhood; for whilft children, they are kept as tender, and are taken as much care of as the children in Denmark : but when the lads are big and ftrong enough to row a boat, and to go a fifhing, they muft then enter upon a fcene of toil and labour, which is very hard, efpecially in the fifhing feafons. Till they attain the fufficient degree of age and ftrength for being capable to go out a fifhing, they are kept within doors, as are alfo the women, and therefore cannot bear much cold or hardfhip. Hence it may be a fubject of furprize, how the men afterwards are able to fuffer fo much, not being brought up thereto from their infancy. The Icelanders, as I faid, are endowed with good bodily ftrength ; but this ftrength continues only from the age of twenty to fifty, at which period it is ufual with them to fall into a decay, by reafon of the various diforders that come upon them, and at laft put an end to their lives. Confumptions and afthmas, the reigning diforders among them, are occafioned chiefly by the many hardfhips they endure at fea in fifhing, and their carelefsnefs of preferving their health. In the latter refpect, they do not mind jumping into the fea to fave their boat from running aground, or receiving damage againft the rocks, and frequently keep on their wet cloaths, even in froft and fnow, without changing any thing. It is very rare to fee any one in this ifland live to a hundred years, or even to eighty. Some may live to that age and enjoy health, but the generality are weak and fickly in their old age, and very few turned of fifty, can boaft of much health. Coughs and confumptions fo afflict them, that none hardly ever wear as well, or have fuch florid complexions as the people of Denmark. In the fifhing feafons, they are obliged to toil very hard ; and at other times they can do nothing, being feveral months in the winter quite idle. Thus by not being conftantly in excercife, the return of labour becomes too heavy and too fatiguing *. Moderate exercife contributes to health, but too hard labour weakens, waftes and fhortens life. As high living

* Mr. Anderfon fays, they lead their lives in ignorance and fimplicity, without any great care, living on a fimple, mean diet, and always employed in bodily exercife.

breeds

breeds difeafes, and makes people old before their time, fo likewife does a too poor and mean food, which cannot yield fufficient
nourifhment to recruit wafted fpirits and ftrength. Plain and fubftantial food moderately ufed, ftrengthens the body, and is productive of long life ; but thefe people cannot even well afford that,
being moftly poor, and fome of them having many children, and
a wife to provide for.   The women are not ufed to any heavy
exercife, or hard labour ; for excepting the hay-harveft, their
other work is chiefly done by them fitting ; fuch as the cleaning
and combing of their wool, fpinning and knitting of gloves,
ftockings, &c. weaving a kind of coarfe cloth, and making their
cloaths, fhoes, and fuch work, as requires no great bodily
ftrength.   As it commonly happens in moft countries, that pea-
fants and labouring people have the beft teeth, fo alfo this is remarkable among the poorer fort of Icelanders, who cannot fpoil
them with high feafoned things, and other dainties, being obliged to content themfelves with a coarfe loaf of rye, which
fcowers their teeth, and leaves them in no want of brufhes or
powders for this purpofe *.   The fame effect they experience in
their dried and well beaten ftock-fifh.   The women are delicate
and chilly, and though their work requires no ftrength, excepting
the hay-harveft, I do not think, that they properly can be
called ftrong and healthy.   In many cafes they ftand in need of
a phyfician.   They have fometimes hard labours, and many of
them die in child-bed for want of the affiftance of fenfible and
experienced midwives †.   In their beft times, they generally keep
their bed unmoved eight days, and many muft even keep it longer, and fuffer a great deal by the ignorance of their midwives ;
and it is not uncommon at thofe times, for a poor woman to be
deprived of her health for ever after.

* Mr. Anderfon fays the Icelanders in general have fine white and found teeth.
† The fame Author fays, the women are as fturdy and as ftrong as the men, and
that they have generally eafy labours, and bathe themfelves as foon as it is over, and
go about their ufual bufinefs.

CHAP.

CHAP. LXXXIV.

Concerning the prevailing difeafes in Iceland.

FROM what has been obferved in the foregoing chapter of the men, when turned of fifty, being troubled with hectic diforders, and the women fubject to very hard labours, which are attended with many accidents ; it may appear, that the Icelanders, as well as the reft of mankind, are liable to various difeafes. They call moft of their difeafes *landfarfot*, which an-fwers what the common people in Denmark call by the general name of *fevers* ; the *landfarfot* being properly not very diffe-rent from a fever in its fymptoms. *Spedalfkhed*, or the leprofy, another difeafe, which many are infected with, is for the moft part hereditary, but not commonly infectious *. This is not the difeafe which goes by that name in Denmark, but rather a fcurvy, of which feveral have been cured by a medicine difcovered by a learned Icelander. Cholics, confumptions, and hypochondriac diforders, are more epidemical among them, and would make good work for a number of phyficians, if the poor people could afford to employ them. The leprofy is the moft prevailing dif-eafe, which continues, as it were, rivetted in them, till they are otherwife worn out with hard labour and age. As it is he-reditary, I don't apprehend that their diet and manner of living, is the caufe of it ; for they are not fo uncleanly a people as they have been reprefented by fome travellers ; and though they are afflicted with various diforders, it cannot be denied, but that they are found in body and conftitution, which are not impaired, but by their many hardfhips and great labour, which at laft expofe them to thofe complicated diforders †. When the Icelanders are

* Mr. Anderfon fays, that fevers and other difeafes are feldom heard of in Iceland, and that there is hardly fuch a thing known as a phyfician or furgeon, their defi-ciency being abundantly compenfated by the many excellent herbs and wholefome mi-neral waters, which the Icelanders continually drink without thinking of their falu-brious qualities. To thefe may be added, the conftant winds that cleanfe and purify the air; the clear, dry and long cold weather, and the innate robuftnefs of the inha-bitants, together with (as it has been before obferved) their excellent digeftion.

† The fame Author fays, that their common difeafes are the cholic and leprofy, which are eafily accounted for by their coarfe and filthy food, and their nafty way of living.

taken ill, they submit themselves to God, and leave nature to help itself, few among them having any medicines, or knowing how to apply them. However, when they feel sickness, they always take some boiled milk made into whey, and set aside the use of tobacco and spirituous liquors, except the patient be so habituated to the same, that he cannot do without them *. The reasons for their not having physicians, may also take place with regard to surgeons, though they frequently stand in need of such, upon account of the misfortunes that sometimes befal them from broken limbs or the like. Their case in these circumstances must be very deplorable, so much the more, as scarce one knows how to apply a proper remedy, for want of which they often perish, or after enduring a deal of pain are miserably cured †. They are not so robust and hardy that nothing can hurt them; for they are human beings, and experience the sensations common to all mankind; and the severe cold and sharp air, are of no service to any of the external hurts and sores they may receive.

C H A P. LXXXV.

How they bring up their children.

WHEN children are put to the breast, they are let to suck as long as is usual in other countries; but the far greater part are brought up by hand. The Icelanders are as tender and as careful of their children, as I ever saw any parents. They have cradles for them, as in other countries, and these of two sorts, some that rock, and others that swing. They give the children the best milk, not skimmed, and never when turned into whey ‡. The milk they are taught to suck out of a horn, in the manner they do in Denmark, to bring them up by hand.

* Mr. Anderson says, if any of them are taken ill, milk only warm from the cow is administred to refresh them, besides a little tobacco to chew, and a large dram of brandy to put their stomach in order.

† The same Author says, they are so hardy and robust, that they do not regard a little hurt; because the greater part of their external hurts soon heal of themselves, probably by reason of the cold and clear air.

‡ He also says, they set their children on the ground, and by them a little vessel with whey, into which they stick a pipe, tied round with thread, or a thick quill, and a bit of bread, if they have it, to strengthen the child: thus when the child wakes, or shews signs of hunger, they turn it about to the vessel, and put the pipe in its mouth, and let it suck as long as it has occasion.

When

When they carry the children to church to be baptized, which is sometimes very remote from their habitations, they generally take such a horn or a phial filled with milk, with a rag tied round for the child to suck through *. In this manner they bring up the children with milk till they are turned of a year old, except there is such a scarcity, that it cannot be had, which happens in some seasons of the year, especially among the poor. Besides the use of cradles, as I before observed, they likewise dress them up in swaddling cloaths, as they do in Denmark, and seldom coat them till they are nine or ten weeks old †. The women carefully tend and nurse them, and carry them about in arms, and in all respects, act the part of tender and fond nurses. The children are all straight and well limbed, hardly any such thing being seen as a cripple among them, and I myself never remarked any hunch-backed, lame, or with other defects, from carelessness in bringing them up.

C H A P. LXXXVI.

Concerning their manner of dressing victuals.

THEY generally boil their fish more than is customary in Denmark, and also boil it in sea-water taken along the coast, which is consistent with reason, and as far as I know better. All their victuals they eat without salt, as before observed, and this too by choice; for though many can afford it, they do not use it for this purpose. Their chief sauce is butter, of which they consume great quantities ‡. They also over boil their meat,

of

* Mr. Anderson says, when they carry their children to be baptized, or to any distance in the country, they dip a rag in whey, and put it in the child's mouth to feed on; but when the children are three quarters of a year old, they make them eat the same food as they do themselves.

† The same Author says, that cradles and swaddling cloaths are things not known to the Icelanders: for as soon as the children are a fortnight old, they put them in a jacket and trowsers, and let them lie crawling on the ground, till they grow big enough to get up and walk. In this miserable manner they are brought up, and hardened from the womb, though no such thing as a cripple is seen among them, or at least very rarely. Hence we may plainly see, how friendly nature alone will operate where a true confidence is reposed, and she is left at liberty; but our Author says, that if there was not proper care taken of them, accidents and hurts would be attended with the same ill consequences as in any other countries.

‡ He here again alledges, that their food is very coarse and mean, their vessels very nasty, and their manner of dressing still worse, and not fit for human creatures.
The

of which they have plenty, and eat more by far than the Danish
farmers, or others of the like sort in many countries. In the
parts that do not abound much in cattle, they exchange fish for
flesh. Undoubtedly here may be found several very poor, as in
all countries, that cannot afford to stock themselves against the
winter, according to wish; but the generality of the farmers
kill ten or twenty sheep for their winter's provision, besides some
neat cattle. All their other victuals are consumed fresh, but
these they preserve in the manner as has been described in the
foregoing part of this treatise. I before observed, that in some
places they have good turf, in others a deal of timber, which
comes floating on the sea to them, and in others little thickets,
but almost every where bushes, furz and heath; so that but few
places are destitute of some sort of fewel, and these particularly
are such tracts of land as project into the sea, or are situate on the
extreme part of the sea coast. Here the inhabitants may be under
some difficulty for want of firing, and the poor must make shift
with sea-weeds, and dried fish-bones *. However these cases are extraordinary, and do not seem as if they deserved to be mentioned. When they kill many sheep together, they most commonly pickle the heads in their syre, a liquor already described, and
as tart as vinegar. These heads are nicely scraped, and boiled
before they pickle them down, which is done in the same manner as in Denmark †. Afterwards for use, they fry them in a
pan. I do not doubt but they may taste tolerably well. The
Icelanders are very fond of any thing that is fat, and some of
the poorer people will eat the melted tallow or fat of their young

The ordinary food among the greater part is a bit of meat, boiled with the heads of
cods, and other fish, which they cut off; though sometimes they afford themselves a
couple of whole cod, which they throw into a pot, pour some sea water on them, and
when boiled a little, take and gobble up without any salt or spice for a relish.

* Mr. Anderson says, they eat neither flesh nor fish while it is fresh catched or killed,
but let it lie by till it begins to stink, otherwise it will not quicken their unpalatable
tongues. The fuel with which they dress their victuals, makes the taste still more
nauseous, few having turf, and fewer wood; so that in general they burn fish, and
other bones, over which they pour the sediment of their oil to make them burn the
better.

† He also says, their most delicate dish is a sheep's head, which they only singe
the wool off, and then put in the hot ashes to bake. When done enough, they eat
it skin and all to the very bones. Our author says, nothing is wanting to this relation, but their eating bones and all, to make downright dogs of them. Mr. Anderson adds, that they are such vast lovers of butter and grease, that they will eat the
very blubber of the whale, and the oil boiled out of the liver.

heifers

heifers or sheep. These poor people having been represented by some travellers and authors, as living in a very bestial manner; I shall here briefly give an exact account of their way of living, and ordinary food.

A great quantity of fresh fish is eaten all over the country, except in the parts that lie too remote from the sea, and the fresh lakes, of which there are but very few, as I before hinted. The quantity of fish dried or cured for keeping, is little in proportion to the great variety of different sorts they get, and must eat fresh. The fish they dry and cure different ways, is chiefly for exportation, and the residue laid up for home consumption, consists mostly of such fish as have changed colour, do not look so clear and white, and are touched by the frost, though in the main, full as well tasted, and as fit for use. They boil their fish generally too much, and use a great deal of butter. The dried or stock-fish, which they eat chiefly in winter, when they cannot get fresh, is well beaten before boiled, and cooked up with a good store of melted butter. They also much use for food the milk of cows and sheep, both raw and boiled, and they prepare of their cows milk their common drink called syre, and in the summer make great quantities to serve them all the year. The curds and sweet milk they feed their servants with, as well as with fish, and also allow them butter. They thicken up their milk with barley, or other grain, and with flour make hasty pudding. They put barley, or other grain, in their broth, for want of herbs and spices. In some places they have cabbage, which they boil in their broth. They use barley in almost all their victuals, and particularly for making a sort of hasty pudding. Their fresh meat they roast or fry, but always first parboil it. Some make use of peas, and rye-meal, to make a dish for the servants. Whatever they boil or fry in their stew-pan, is always quite fresh, and they rather over boil all their fish and flesh-meat, because it goes very much against them to eat any thing that is not thoroughly done. Their kitchen utensils they generally have from Copenhagen. Their pots and kettles are of iron, brass or copper, which they keep neat and sweet. All of them dress their victuals very clean, except some few, who, no doubt, are as nasty as elsewhere, but a whole country should

F f
not

not be vilified, much lefs involved in the fame fcandal on their account. Thofe that have been abroad, and at Copenhagen, drefs their victuals in the Danifh manner, and live as nice as folks do there; others learn from them, and in all other refpects, every one lives according to his inclinations and circumftances.

CHAP. LXXXVII.

Concerning the fcarcity of bread.

AS no hufbandry is followed at prefent in Iceland, bread muft be fcarce, and of confequence not fo univerfally the food of the meaner fort as in Denmark. However, it is not fo very fcarce, but that they may have it, and lay up a provifion, each according to his abililies *. I before mentioned the quantity of bread and meal imported into each harbour, which is from 400 to 1000 tun † of flour, one third whereof is baked into bread, and though not fufficient for their daily fubfiftence, yet they cannot be faid to be entirely without it. For celebrating feafts, weddings, and publick meetings, they are always provided with bread; and thofe that have lived at Copenhagen, not doing well without it, take care to have it all the year round. It is no faving to them, in not having a fufficiency of bread for their families: their houfekeeping is the dearer for it, and their manner of feeding their fervants, &c. is fo expenfive, that it would not anfwer even in Denmark. Each fervant man is allowed to the amount of ten pounds of dried fifh, and three pounds and a half of butter per week: but none are thus portioned except thofe that are fent on journies, or to the fouthward to fifh. Such as continue at home, have a portion of fifh and butter every day, or have frefh fifh, and fometimes flefh-meat, broth, peas, and the like. The Icelanders by not having a fufficiency of bread, are obliged to ufe a deal of dried fifh, but not to eat it as bread with other food. This fifh is firft well beaten, and eaten without boiling, with butter like a piece of bread. Spread over

* Mr. Anderfon fays, that the greater part of them, not being in circumftances to buy the meal which the Danifh merchants import, are obliged to live without bread.

† A tun is eight fkiepp, or bufhels.

in this manner with butter, it has a very good relifh, efpecially
dried trout, whitings, &c. * Some of our Danifh civil officers
liked it fo well, that they ufed it on their journies, and eat it
with pleafure. The wild corn that grows in fome places, efpecially in the diftrict of Skaftefield, though not in any great
quantity, makes very good flour and bread. It is very nourifh-
ing, and the Icelanders will not exchange a tun of it for a tun of
Danifh †. It fhoots up in deep fand, where no grafs will grow.
In fome places it ftands very thin, in others pretty thick, and
runs up two foot and a half high. The ears are long, and it
grows much like the wheat in Denmark. As the Icelanders have
no good mills to grind their corn, they dry it too much before
the fire, even burn it a little, which makes the bread blacker
than the rye bread is in Denmark.

C H A P. LXXXVIII.

Concerning their drink.

THE Icelanders are fond of clear water; but the water is
not good every where, neither are every where mineral
waters found ‡. The water that runs from Jokells none drink
of, being very thick, black and ftinking, as I elfewhere have
obferved. But though they love water, their chief liquor is
fyre, of which in fummer they fill up many barrels to laft all
the winter. Thofe that keep a good ftock of cattle, make it
for fale. It is drank at firft without any adulteration; but
when it grows old, it becomes too four, and they then mix
water with it. This liquor agrees very well with them. As
no corn is cultivated in the country, beer confequently muft be
very fcarce, yet it may be had, and thofe that go to the trading
towns or factories about bufinefs, are always fure to find fome,
of which they buy a certain quantity to indulge themfelves

* Mr. Anderfon fays, that inftead of bread, they eat dried ftock-fifh, and fuch as
is not faleable. They only beat it a little, and eat it with butter; but when they
have no butter, they take blubber, train or tallow, and fpread it thereon.
† The fame Author fays, there is a wild corn that fhoots up fpontaneoufly among
the grafs, which they make bread of, but foreigners cannot eat it.
‡ He alfo fays, they praife the water that runs from the top of the mountains,
which is nothing but the ice and fnow melted by the fun.

with

with at home. Some of them lay in feveral barrels at a time, and make ufe of it fparingly all the year round. Thofe that have been at Copenhagen, cannot do without it. They import malt and hops, which they brew themfelves, and they may have beer very well all the year round; but for this purpofe they muft brew every third or fourth week *. Though they have no cellar, yet the beer does not freeze more than it would at Copenhagen, where they have them very good and convenient. The hardeft frofts fcarce freeze more than the cock, which is rendered pliable, by holding hot coals under it before the beer will run, and fometimes only by fetting a pan of coals in the room. Some of the people keep French wine, both red and white, particularly the minifters, who ufe it for the facrament. Generally fpeaking, there is not a more fober people than the Icelanders. I knew fome, and even of the more common fort, that do not chufe to drink brandy, and feveral that drink it very moderately. There may be a few, as in other countries, who are very fond of it. When they come to the factories about bufinefs, they then indulge themfelves with brandy, and other liquors †. A merchant or ftranger, on firft coming to thefe places, may be induced to deem them a drunken, beaftly people; and I myfelf was almoft of that opinion, till I came into the country to be better acquainted with their manner of living. It is certain, that at the factories which they refort to but once a year, they drink brandy to excefs; for it comes but feldom in their way, and is as great a treat to them, as a bottle of Hungary or Cape wine to a merchant. But as this happens only occafionally, they cannot be called drunkards, much lefs compared with thofe that are continually craving brandy, and drink themfelves drunk whenever they can lay hold of it. When one confiders the fmall quantity of brandy that is imported for 80,000 people, it is plain there cannot be many drunkards among them. In each factory

---

* Mr. Anderfon fays, that by not having cellars, they cannot keep their ale for any time, on account of the fevere cold.

† The fame Author fays, that fome of the fubftantial people among them lay up French wine at the factories for their own ufe; but as they put it in dirty veffels, and fometimes in thofe that have had four whey, and even train oil, without firft cleaning them, the wine turns foul and ftinking. He adds, that in general, brandy is the liquor they are fond of, and that by it, young and old, men and women, fhamefully get drunk.

there

there may be a fcore of drunken, idle fellows, always begging of brandy, or expending all they get on it; but what are fo few to the reft, who are very abftemious, and on their account, fhould not receive the charaéter of drunkards.   I never faw, nor heard of the women getting drunk.   When they come to the factories, I have feen them refufe brandy, and inftead of it take a glafs of mafs wine, which is the name they give Frenoh wine. Sometimes on taking their children with them to the factory, a father will give his fon a drop of brandy, that he may tafte fomething good, as he calls it, in the world ; for it is the next precious liquor to wine they know of, and the poor children have no other opportunity ever to tafte it *.   The generality cannot lay out much on this commodity at the factories, having many other things to purchafe, as meal, timber, fifhing-lines, iron, cloth, and a variety of other neceffaries.   The better fort lay in a little ftock of brandy, which ferves them all the year ; but thofe that are drunkards, cannot afford to ftock themfelves with it, and if they do, they cannot let it alone till all is gone.

C H A P.   LXXXIX.

Concerning their drefs.

THE Icelanders are contented in procuring the implements of drefs out of their own manufactures, which fhews wifdom and prudence in them, and it were to be wifhed, that other nations did the fame.   Their outfide apparel is generally a coarfe bays, which they call *vadmel.*   The women for the greater part have petticoats and aprons of coloured cloth, of which fome thoufand ells are fold every year.   This cloth is not fuperfine ; but they have it of different goodnefs, all of Danifh manufacture.   The better fort, both men and women, wear cloth jackets.   As for the lawyers, and thofe in civil employ-ments, they drefs in the modern fafhion, with full fuits lined

* Mr. Anderfon fays, that in all their dangers both by fea and land, brandy is their principal comfort, and the main point they have in view.   It encourages them to labour, that they may get fomething to purchafe fo precious a liquor.   When they have attained their wifh, and provided themfelves with brandy, on the arrival of the Danifh fhips, they never leave off drinking till all is gone ; for while any is left, they can do no bufinefs.

with

with filk, and in every refpect as genteel as at Copenhagen. The
cloaths of the common people are made like thofe of feafaring
men, namely, jackets and wide breeches, or trowfes, though
fometimes they wear a coat made in the Danifh fafhion. They
have befides a great coat, which they call *hempe*, and wear in
the winter to go to church in, or on a journey. The women
wear petticoats, jackets and aprons of woollen cloth or bays,
which they call *vadmel*, and over which they wear a kind of
wide coat, with narrow fleeves, that reaches down to their wrifts.
Thefe coats or gowns, are a hands breadth fhorter than the petticoats ; they are always black, and are called by the name of
hempe, which is the fame the mens. great coats go by. Sometimes they are faced with black velvet, and fometimes the work
on them refembles *point de la reine*, which is very neat, and looks
well. Thofe that are rich, have wrought filver and gilt buckles,
or clafps, which are only faftened on for fhow or ornament. The
petticoats and aprons which are coloured, are bordered round and
down the edges with flips of coloured velvet, or coloured filk
ribbands, or a filk braid at the tie of their apron. Three great
filver philligre worked buttons, and generally gilt, are fixed before. The poorer women have them of brafs. The apron is
faftened to a belt, fet all round with filver buttons, or of brafs,
according to their circumftances, and clafped before with a clafp
of the fame metal and workmanfhip. Their jackets are always
made to fit neat and clofe to the waift, with narrow fleeves down
to their wrifts, and are laced in all the feams with coloured velvet or ribbands, and faced down before with filk. On each
fleeve near the wrift, are four or fix buttons of filver or brafs ;
and round the neck a ftiff cape is worn about three fingers
breadth, which ftands erect, and under it the wide coat is
made to go. This cape is covered with handfome filk or
black velvet, and a gold or filver braid round it. About their
head they tie a coarfe white linen handkerchief, and over that
another finer, formed like a tuft on the top of the head, and a
foot and a half high. Over this they place a filk handkerchief,
or the poorer fort a cotton one, which is tied under the chin.
This kind of head-drefs is worn by all women, whether fingle
or married, and round their necks they have ufually another filk

or

or cotton handkerchief*. In short, their dress much resembles what is met with in old pictures, and monuments in churches, except the head-dress, of which I have not remarked any thing similar in any other country. The young girls wear caps, but when grown up, they change them for those high heads. The richer sort have a deal of finery about them, consisting of silver and gilt philligree work, which they most admire. Some large buttons of that sort of work, with coloured stones set in them, and fastened to their fillet, are worn a little above their forehead. A bride on her wedding-day, wears a crown of silver under the white linnen tuft that stands up so high on their heads, and on this occasion is used instead of the silk handkerchief worn at other times. They wear also two silver chains, the one hanging down behind, and the other in the same manner on the breast. The *hempe* or great coat, is never worn during these solemnities. To the bottom of another chain, which hangs down before, a box of perfumes is fastened, with several partitions, and open on both sides. It is very often shaped like a heart or a cross. I have seen some of them of gold. Several of the Iceland ladies have trinkets to the amount of three or four hundred rixdollars; and indeed their dress is vastly neat and pretty. The men and womens shoes, which most commonly are all made by the women, are of their ox's hides, or for want of them, of sheepskins, which they dress themselves, by only scraping the hair off, and afterwards drying them. To set about making the shoes, they first soak the leather in water, and when duly prepared, they go through all the different operations, and seldom fail to fit them exactly to the feet, but scarce ever trouble themselves about fixing heels to them. Their shirts and shifts are usually made of thin bays or flannel, though a great many have them of coarse linen †. Their fishing garb is made of sheep-skin, which they put over their other cloaths to keep off the wet, and which

* Mr. Anderson says, that their dress and habitations are all of a piece with their eating and drinking; but that the unmarried women wear handkerchiefs round their chins, to distinguish them from the married.

† The same Author says, that the men and women wear linen shirts and shifts, or properly stockings and breeches of one piece, which reach on the men above the navel, but not up to the navel on the women, over which they have other breeches and a jacket of *vadmel*, or coarse bays, or else of sheep-skin.

they

they daub with fifh liver to foften them ; but they pull them off
as foon as they come afhore.

CHAP. XC.

Concerning their habitations.

AT the entrance of their houfes, a long narrow paffage is
formed about fix foot wide, with crofs beams, a covering,
and fome holes on the fide of the door to admit light fufficient
for the paffage. In thefe holes are fometimes panes of glafs,
but moft commonly a thin fkin or bladder ftretched upon a
frame, which affords a tolerable light. There are fhutters for
thefe and other windows, in rainy or fnowy weather. At the
end of this paffage is the entrance into their common room,
which is generally twenty-four or twenty-eight feet long, and
about twelve or fixteen broad. Here the women fit and drefs
their wool, fpin, and do other neceffaries for the family. At
the further end of this room is generally a bed-chamber for the
mafter and miftrefs of the houfe, and in the loft over it, the
children and maid-fervants generally lie. On each fide of the
aforefaid paffage, are two rooms, with doors in the paffage. The
one is ufed for a dining-room, the other a dairy, the third
for the kitchen, and the fourth, which is juft by the outer door,
for the men fervants to lie in, or ftrangers of that fex, who are
a travelling. This whole building confifts of fix rooms, and
but one ftreet or outer door. Holes are made in the feveral
rooms to tranfmit the light, and as in the paffage, are covered
with panes of glafs, or with a fkin or bladder. In the large
common room, moft people have a couple of fmall windows,
in order to fee to work the better. They have alfo frequently
a room built on one fide, clofe to' that appropriated for the men
fervants, which they call their ftate-room, where they receive vi-
fits. A bed is fixed therein, and a door that leads directly in
or out without paffing through the houfe, and another door into the fervants bed-chamber, through which the people of the
houfe pafs and repafs, without being obliged to go about. They
have warehoufes detached from the dwelling-houfe, to keep their
fifh, and winter provifion in; their horfe furniture, their imple-

ments

ments for hay-making, &c. near this they have another little
building, which is their fmith's-fhop. Here they make all their
tools and tackle of iron and wood *. At a little diftance ftand
their barns and ftables, and one, two, three or four fheep-folds.
In one of thefe they keep the lambs by themfelves. Their hay
is ftacked up about fix foot fquare, and a paffage left between
each ftack, and covered with turf, in a fhelving manner, for
the rain to run off, by which means their hay is well preferved.
Their common room, bed-chamber and vifiting room, are generally wainfcotted, and have a loft over them, where their chefts,
wearing apparel, &c. are kept. Thefe upper apartments have
alfo windows, two or three panes high; but the other buildings
without either lofts or windows, have only holes for the light, as
I before obferved, with a pane, or the thin fkin † taken out of
the ftomach of animals, and ftretched on a frame whilft warm,
after which it becomes very tranfparent, and admits the light.
Their furniture is not any way coftly, and confifts chiefly of
beds, and their vadmel or bays, which ferves them for making
pillows and bedding of. They have plenty of feathers, but fome
of their common fervants lie very wretchedly, as often the poor
and mean people in Denmark do. They have tables, ftools,
benches, chefts, and other neceffary utenfils for a houfe. Thofe
of better rank and fortune, have their habitations well furnifhed
with looking-glaffes, and every thing that is requifite in a genteel way. As there is a great fcarcity of timber in the ifland,
and as building materials muft be bought of the company, which
confequently prove very expenfive, the inhabitants are obliged to
proceed to work in the moft frugal manner they can. They
therefore lay a foundation of large ftones, upon which they

---

* Mr. Anderfon fays, their houfes for the fake of ftrength as well as warmth, are
funk into the ground, and are feldom above feven foot high, in length about twenty-
four or twenty-eight feet, and in breadth not more than when a tall man ftanding in
the middle and ftretching out his arms, may reach the fide walls, which makes
them about fix foot wide. Along the fide of the wall, they build a loofe flight covering, high enough for the cattle to be fheltered in during the winter. The fame alfo
ferves for the fervants to lie in; for they only lay a little ftraw on the ground, on
which they lie quite naked and cover themfelves with a piece of bays, which is fometimes lined with a fheep-fkin. In this manner they lie, the one's head againft the
other's feet, or perhaps a board put between, to feparate thofe that do not belong to
each other.

† Tunicas allantoidas.

H h   erect

erect the frame-work of their building. The crofs beams and joifts they faften the beft way they can. Between the timber work, they make a wall of clay and ftones, and afterwards lay the rafters for the top, which are but fmall. The beft houfes are covered with boards, which are nailed an inch or two over one another, for the rain to run off without running through. Meaner houfes have furze and twigs a top inftead of boards, and are covered with turf. The walls are of ftones, and earth, or clay, with grafs or turf between, which befides is laid over all the pofts and beams, and thus renders the walls very firm, ftrong, and well bound at the foundation. They are ufually made four foot thick, and run up flanting, that at top they may be about three foot in thicknefs. This fort of walls makes warm habitations, and keeps out equally the heat in fummer, and the cold in winter; fo that in this laft feafon, they have no occafion to keep great fires, though fome in feveral parts are provided with ftoves. The foundation of the houfes built after this manner, is even with the ground, or raifed a little higher. When the walls are all green, they appear like fo many hillocks. All farmers have not fuch large habitations as defcribed, nor are they furnifhed with fo many feparate buildings, though many have much larger and finer: but in fuch a general defcription as this, it is much the better way to keep between extremes, by exhibiting that which is more univerfal, as has been reprefented in the defcription of a good farm-houfe, the proper model, for conveying the jufteft idea of the place, whereas by delineating a miferable hut, this idea, or any thing refulting from it, could be no more anfwered, than it would by difplaying the magnificence of his Majefty's feat at Beffefted, or of fome of the bifhops and lawyers houfes, or thofe of the civil magiftrates, and fome of the inferior clergy. Thefe houfes are built of brick, like thofe in Denmark, and the bifhop's feat at Holum, confifts of fifty feparate buildings, befides twelve ftables, or houfes for cattle; but fuch are far from being a rule for the buildings in general throughout the ifland. I have been at feveral other farms, which are like villages, with many feparate buildings, but all fuch buildings belong to one and the fame farm.

CHAP.

C H A P. XCI.

Concerning their genius, and natural difpofition of mind.

THE annals of this country fhew, that in ancient times they were a warlike people, having in their inteftine broils made great flaughter among themfelves. They are far from being a daftardly race, as fome authors have reprefented them; for it is well known that they made fome figure in a military life, and have been raifed to the command of fortreffes. However, as this country cannot fpare many of its inhabitants, and as fortunately for them, it is too remote for officers to come and mufter up a body of recruits, few of them for thefe reafons have been employed in the military way. In the fea fervice fome of them have been promoted to the command of Dutch veffels; and indeed, they feem beft adapted to a feafaring life, being trained up to it almoft from their infancy. The many ingenious Icelanders fo eminent in the literary world, is a ftrong inftance of their genius and good natural parts, and that they are not of a flavifh abject difpofition. Every year fome of their felect youth are fent to the univerfity at Copenhagen, where they have conftant opportunities of exhibiting their genius and capacity, which are difcovered to be very remote from betraying an abject fpirit, the reverfe rather appearing in them, together with fuch a fpirit of emulation for excelling others, that feldom or ever a dull perfon is remarked among them: and even in general, the common people have keen cunning heads, and a deal of mother wit. As moft other nations, they have a ftrong propenfity to their native place, though one might think they would find more pleafure in other countries. Perhaps in this refpect, the hankering after home prevails more among the northern people than any others. However, many eftablifh themfelves at Copenhagen, and in other foreign countries, when they have fettled in any certain bufinefs; and among thefe may be feen profeffors, rectors, feafaring people, goldfmiths, and mafters in a variety of handicraft occupations. The Icelanders complain that their countrymen who go abroad, and learn many things, whereby they might be of vaft fervice to them, fcarce

ever

ever return *. I fhall not undertake to examine, whether this complaint be well founded : fome few undoubtedly do, and at the bifhop's feat of Holum, there is now an Icelander, that underftands the art of printing to perfection. He learnt it at Copenhagen, and fince travelled about in foreign parts, and was fent for from Dantzick to come home. The Icelanders are alfo as induftrious as moft people in their feveral occupations, never neglecting, or omitting any thing that ought to be done. I have feen them row out to fea fifty or fixty times, and perhaps they did not bring home in all above fixteen or twenty fifh. The general failing of the common people in moft countries, proceeds from their being wedded to old cuftoms, which they will not retract, unlefs upon the profpect of very confiderable advantage †. This is the cafe of the Icelanders, though I prefume, they are rather more cautious than obftinate, in rejecting their old cuftoms ; for I muft confefs, that I found them fond of feeing curiofities, and of improving themfelves, as alfo very ready to imitate, very handy at making any thing, and very expert in turning things to advantage.

C H A P. XCII.

Whether they delight in learning any thing.

ICELAND has produced Thormodus Thorfæus, and Arnas Magnæus, befides feveral other illuftrious men. Some Iceland ftudents are now at the univerfity, and far from being reputed inferior to any, on the contrary, generally excel, few being ever bad, or even middling among them. It is not at Copenhagen alone that they are thus found ingenious, the people in the country are confpicuous for like abilities ; they prefently learn any thing they are put to, and not fimply what they have

---

* Mr. Anderfon fays, that their poor diet and fatiguing life, which only exercifes their body, cannot elevate their mental faculties, or ferve to make any improvements in them, and that being naturally of a daftardly difpofition, they are very unfit for foldiers.

† The fame Author fays, that they are a very licentious people, which is owing to the too great liberty they enjoy, whereby they become ftupid and perverfe, and are fo bigotted to their own cuftoms, that though they are fhewed fhorter and better methods, yet they reject all, and purfue their own old and obftinate ways.

been

been brought up to from their early youth *. It is not the few only that have been abroad, who learned to be penmen and accomptants, and to work ingeniously in gold, silver, brass, and the like; but even the greater part of the inhabitants, who never were out of the island, write very well. Among the learned are some excellent writers, and among the clergy and the people in general, more write well than in Denmark. Those that go to Copenhagen, carry all those good qualifications along with them. There are not, it is true, so many good accomptants as writers, yet several may be found, who never were out of the country. The Icelanders that apply themselves to any particular science in Denmark, generally become masters of it. Copenhagen can afford several instances in this respect: even in Iceland, many very ingenious men having taught themselves without the instructions of a master, work in silver and brass, and make philligre buttons and buckles for the women. They are also ingenious carpenters, joiners, and smiths. In short, they exercise themselves in all manner of trades, and some, by applying themselves entirely to one particular branch, become at last perfect masters in it. They are very fond of taking notice of for imitation, or contriving themselves such new tools and instruments as are handy and convenient for their work; and indeed this may appear from the great improvements they have made therein, and at the same time, may be a convincing proof of the delight and pleasure they take in edification †. They calculate time by the sun, or stars, when visible, but if not, they then adjust this point by the tide, which is always regular. Thus not counting time by the clock or hour, as one, two, three, or four o'clock, which they know nothing of, they have particular names for every hour and half in the day in their own language, as for instance, noon, midnight, midevening, broad day, &c.

* Mr. Anderson says, that a propensity to arts and sciences is not in the least observable among them, yet he does not suppose, that they are naturally quite stupid, and not able to comprehend any thing. Some learned men have appeared in their country, and such of them as have travelled, distinguished themselves as very ingenious artisans.

† The same Author allows them to have some ingenuity; for with very aukward and bad tools, he says, they notwithstanding complete the various things they have occasion for. He also says, they have no calculation of time, and only regulate themselves herein by the ebb and flood, or the sun, when they can see it.

C H A P.

CHAP. XCIII.

Concerning their occupations.

HAVING before often obferved, that the chief occupation of the Icelanders is fifhing, or breeding of cattle, and having alfo defcribed their manner of fifhing, and curing fifh, I fhall here only add, an account of their manner of building boats *. In the diftrict of Guldbringe, they build their boats of oak, but in other parts moft commonly of fir, which by experience they find to be full as ftrong and as durable as oak, and attended with much lefs expence. In fome places they are made fmall, and only for two men to row in, though even thefe will carry a cargo of 120 fine large cod ; but for the generality, they are built in moft parts big enough to be rowed by four, fix, eight, and fometimes twenty men ; and the fmall ones are hardly feen any where but at Guldbringe, and about Hvalfiorden. In the diftricts of Rangervalle and Skaftefield, where the coaft is open and fandy, they are obliged to drag their boats a great way up the fhore, that they may lie fecure and fafe from the waves of the fea †. Here alfo they have the largeft boats. In other parts of the ifland, they have but a fhort way to drag their boats, in order to fave them from receiving any damage ; for the coaft is no where fo flat as in the former diftricts. The fort of anchor they there ufe, confifts of a couple of fticks run crofs-ways through a heavy ftone. I have feen the fame in other places, and was affured, that they hold very faft to the ground, and that the fifhermen are not afraid of their holding, even out at fea, if they have good ftrong ropes or cables, which generally break before the ftone gives way. Whenever they make a fhort voyage with their boats, and have got their cargo in, if a contrary wind happens, they will lie feveral days at anchor, rather than drag their boats afhore.

* Mr. Anderfon fays, that their boats ufually built of thin oak boards, are fo light, that two men can carry them on their fhoulders with eafe.

† The fame Author fays, that having neither ropes nor anchors to faften their boats with, they drag them very far up the fhore, to keep them from the waves, and to prevent their being carried away, or dafhed to pieces.

CHAP.

C H A P. XCIV.

Concerning their cattle-trade.

IN the former part, where a defcription was given of the manner of breeding cattle, the trade carried on with them, and
the fifheries, I fhewed that in fome places, breeding of cattle
and grazing, was the chief bufinefs of the inhabitants, who generally fend their cattle up the country, and keep people to look
after them.   The greateft part of the ifland is well ftocked with
cattle, efpecially northward and eaftward, where many farmers
have from two hundred to five hundred fheep, which they turn
out at certain feafons, and at others keep within folds. The
fheep, which give milk are fuffered to run about near the houfes,
and are feparated from the reft.   Two or three times a year they
are all driven together, (which the Icelanders call Soyde-retter) to
be fent to the factories, and there fold *.   Each of thefe particulars I have already fet forth at large.

C H A P. XCV.

Concerning the Icelander's tannery.

TANNING is performed in a very indifferent, or imperfect
manner in Iceland, the inhabitants being in want of bark,
and other neceffaries for this purpofe. However, as obliged
to make the beft fhift they can, they fcrape the wool or hair
off with a fharp knife on their knees, which they do very expeditioufly, and afterwards wafh, clean, and dry the fkins, or
hides. To make the leather tough, and of fome confiftence,
they tread it for a confiderable time with their feet in whey or
falt water.   When afhore or at home, they wear no fort of leather but in their fhoes; but when they go to fea to fifh, they
have a jacket, breeches and ftockings, made of leather, which
keep off the rain and fea water, and prevent their being wet

* Mr, Anderfon fays, that the trade with their cattle in general, does not give
them much trouble, and that in particular, the inhabitants of Weftmanöe turn out
their fheep on the fmall neighbouring iflands, where there is good ftore of grafs, and
from whence, as they cannot get away, they are eafily caught.

through,

through, which muſt happen, if they had not on ſuch a covering *. This outſide leather dreſs they lubricate with fiſh-liver,
and train-oil, that the water may neither adhere, nor be ſoaked
in; but the ſmell preceding therefrom is ſo diſagreeable, that
they never appear before the factors, or any of their betters in
this garb, and uſually take care to ſtrip it off, as ſoon as they
come aſhore. They have a way of giving a blackiſh colour to
the ox hide which they uſe for ſaddles, and horſe furniture; and
though there is nothing of art in it, but meer labour, it is notwithſtanding more durable than the Daniſh: but the ſaddles and
horſe furniture they make up themſelves, are not ſo tough and
pliable as the Daniſh, though they greaſe them with train-oil,
which daubs the cloaths, and is otherwiſe very diſagreeable *.

C H A P. XCVI.

Concerning ſome other of their employments.

WHEN they have nothing elſe to do, the men, women,
and children, eſpecially in winter, work at the cleaning,
combing, twining and ſpinning of wool. Their manner of
weaving is much out of character; for inſtead of having their
weaving benches or frames in an horizontal poſition, as we have
them in Denmark, theirs are perpendicular, or upright, and ſo
inconvenient, that they cannot weave above half a yard a day
of their coarſe bays, or as they call it vadmel, whereby it may
appear how inconſiderable the earnings are *per diem*, of thoſe
who in this reſpect are obliged to get a livelihood by journey-
work. Of late ſome Daniſh weavers came among them, and
the Icelanders begin to imitate them ſo well, that it is probable
this manufacture will in time gain conſiderable improvements, ſo
much the more, as his Daniſh majeſty has alſo ſet up ſeveral
weaving frames, and ordered ingenious maſters from Denmark

---

* Mr. Anderſon ſays, that their way of dreſſing leather is only by laying the hide
on their naked knee, and ſcraping the hair off with a knife, after which, it is fit for
any purpoſe they want it. He adds, that all the leather and ſkins they uſe are greaſed
every fourth or fifth day with fiſh-liver, which makes them tough, but at the ſame
time of ſo offenſive a ſmell, that no merchant or factor can ſpeak to them, or endure
to have them come near them.

† He alſo ſays, that the Icelanders live amidſt perpetual ill ſmells, and a kind of
hoggiſh filthineſs.

to go over, by whom the natives being inſtructed in the proper methods of weaving, cannot fail of ſucceeding with regularity and good order, in this uſeful branch of buſineſs. As hitherto they have had no fulling-mills, it muſt be imagined that they have a deal of trouble in fulling and milling all the woollen goods made in the country, ſuch as jackets, breeches, ſtockings, mittins, &c. and indeed it is ſo; for when they ſet about fulling, they have no other inſtrument for this purpoſe than a caſk, or a barrel, with both bottoms ſtruck out, into which, having put the woollen goods to be milled, two perſons place themſelves on the ground over-againſt each other, and with their feet, go through the operation in the caſk or barrel. Small things they full upon a table againſt their breaſt, but both ways are very toilſome, and attended with great trouble. As for gloves and mittins, they put them on when they are going to ſea, and after dipping them in the ſea-water, they mill them as they row upon their hands, without any farther trouble. Thoſe near the hot wells, mill their things therein, and beſides a quick diſpatch, make them much whiter. In fulling breeches and ſtockings, they are often put on, and the parties rock themſelves about with them, by which means they have contracted a habit of perpetually rocking and moving their limbs, though they have nothing on or under them that wants milling. The women waſh their things generally in urine, uſing neither ſoap nor lye, which are too expenſive, and muſt be imported. However, they waſh their things tolerably well, though I muſt ſuppoſe, not to the liking of all perſons. Thoſe that have been in Copenhagen, import ſoap, and waſh as they do there. In point of dying, which many of them underſtand, they extract verdigreaſe with urine, from copper veſſels, whereby they dye their woollen yarn, and weave pretty ſtriped woollen ſtuffs of various colours.

K k   C H A P.

C H A P. XCVII.

Concerning their manner of merchandizing.

WHEN the Icelander brings his goods for sale to the factory, the merchant does not take them of him *bonâ fide*,
till every thing is separately examined, and passes through his
hands, so that whatever is found unmerchantable, is set aside.
Sometimes, in such great quantities, some indifferent things may
slip in, but the Icelander does not deserve to be blamed; it is
the merchant's fault, if he does not pay attention to what he
buys *. The new map published with this treatise, points out
all the harbours in the island. The fish-harbours lie south and
west, and the flesh-harbour north and east; but in some of the
harbours, as Oreback and Stikkefsholm, both flesh and fish are
delivered †. These harbours were farmed out to merchants at
Copenhagen, and the merchant, who took a fish-harbour, was
also obliged to have a flesh one: but in 1733, a company being
erected, and a charter granted, to trade to all the harbours in
the island, the merchants keep their factors and factories at
every harbour, and send their ships with super-cargoes, though
sometimes one ship will touch at two different harbours, according as the company may think necessary. Besides these, there
are factors or merchants at each harbour, that go with the ships,
and it is they that purchase from the natives their commodities,
on the company's account, and give them other merchandize in
return, or pay them in ready money, all according to a printed
tax-price, by which they must regulate themselves on both sides,
this regulation having taken place ever since the year 1733. The
whole island with Westmanöerne, is all farmed out to this company, and the factors at the flesh-harbours, fix the days for the

---

* Mr. Anderson expresses great surprize, with regard to the deceit and cunning of
these people, who put in practice so much artifice, that one must take the greatest
care and caution imaginable to deal with them.
† The same Author, in order to give a perfect description of their trade, says,
that it is necessary to understand, that the island has fourteen fishing harbours, and
eight flesh, the former lying north and east, and the latter south and west, and that
these harbours being farmed out to merchants at Copenhagen, those that take a fish-
harbour, must also take a flesh one. Our author says the harbours are now otherwise
disposed of.

farmers

farmers to deliver their sheep from each district, and contrive to dispatch the ships as quick as possible. The cattle are slaughtered for the factors about the latter end of August, or beginning of September; but the Icelanders kill none for their own use till the middle of October, at which time the cattle are fattest and finest, and have sensibly more tallow than when they are killed in August *. The Icelanders slaughter all the cattle for the factors, and have the head and offals for their trouble. The meat is salted down by the company's people, and is cut as at Copenhagen, chiefly in large pieces. The skins of the sheep are sprinkled on the flesh-side with salt, and being laid together two by two, are rolled up, and tied very tight together, and thus are pretty well preserved. The tallow is melted and poured into firkins or barrels. The factors take all the good dried fish, consisting of large, small, and middling cod and ling, according to the tax as before observed, though of the latter but few are catched or brought to market. At the fishing harbours, the factors also buy up the train-oil. Woollen goods are chiefly brought to the flesh-harbours, though some are delivered indiscriminately at all.

C H A P. XCVIII.

Concerning accompts and payments.

IN Iceland, no other money is current than specie † and Danish crowns, and all accounts are adjusted according to the number of fish. Two pounds of fish, are worth two skillings specie, and forty-eight fish make one rixdollar specie. A Danish crown, according to the tax, is computed to be the value of thirty fish, a half-crown of fifteen, an half specie of twenty-four, and a quarter of twelve, which is the smallest money current in Iceland. In this manner all payments are regulated by fish, and whatever comes to less than the value of twelve fish, can-

---

* Mr. Anderson says, the merchants buy the cattle the latter end of August, or beginning of September, at which time the cold coming in, and the grass changing, and therefore not so nourishing, the cattle of consequence begin to fall off.

† Specie is bank money, and consists of all pieces of a whole, half, quarter or eighth rixdollar. A rixdollar specie is about 3 s. 6 d. sterling

not

not be paid in money, but muſt either in fiſh, or roll tobacco, an ell of which is equal to a fiſh; ſo that fiſh and tobacco ſerve there inſtead of ſmall coin. The largeſt weight, called vette, is forty fiſh, or eighty pounds, equal to five liſpound in Denmark; the next to this, called föring, is five fiſh, or ten pounds, and the ſmalleſt, or ſingle pound, is computed equal to half a fiſh; for one fiſh is generally of two pounds weight.

C H A P. XCIX.

Concerning the goods they export.

THE commodities they export are dried fiſh, ſalted lambs fleſh, ſome beef, butter, train-oil, a great quantity of tallow, woollen goods, as coarſe and fine bays, or vadmel jackets, ſtockings and gloves, raw wool, ſheep-ſkins, young lamb-ſkins, foxes ſkins of various colours, edder-down and feathers, and formerly ſulphur, but now not taken any more from them: theſe are the chief commodities of this country.

C H A P. C.

Concerning the goods they import.

THE goods imported to Iceland are timber, fiſhing-lines, tobacco, bread, horſe-ſhoes, brandy, wine, ſalt, coarſe linen, a ſmall quantity of ſilk, and a few other things people in good circumſtances may have occaſion for in their families. All theſe commodities are to be imported only by the Danes, who for this purpoſe erected a company, and have a charter from their ſovereign for the excluſive privilege; ſo that no other nation is allowed to trade there. Whatever the Icelander takes, he makes a return for in his own goods, which if not ſufficient, the balance is paid in the above-mentioned money.

CHAP. CI.

Concerning their weights and meafures.

THE weights of the Icelanders agree with the Danifh, pound and pound alike, except that they have no lifpound and fhip-pound, theirs being confined to pounds, förings and vette. Ten pound is a föring, and eighteen förings make a vette, equal to five lifpounds in Denmark. Their ell is fomething fhorter than the Danifh, and agrees with that of Hamburgh *. But as this ell is the only meafure they ufe that agrees with the Hamburg, it cannot with any juft foundation from thence be inferred, when weights and other meafures are different, that the Hamburghers were the firft that eftablifhed trade among them. Certain it is, that they once traded to this ifland, and inftituted a fociety or company, fometimes called by the name of the fociety or company of Iceland traders, and fometimes by the title of *lurendreyers :* but the prefent company eftablifhed at Copenhagen, will now neither fuffer the Hamburghers, nor any other nation to trade there. They pay an annual acknowledgment to the king, and having by a charter granted them, the fole privilege of this trade, they cannot allow interlopers to intercept their profits. The Dutch a few years ago, had two of their fhips confifcated, which they fent to the northward in the diftrict of Skagefiord, with contraband goods ; and fome time before, had five fhips taken from them by a Danifh man of war, which were condemned at Copenhagen as lawful prizes †. Ever fince, foreigners have not attempted to trade to this place, though I fuppofe the Dutch, notwithftanding thefe rebuffs, ftill now and then touch at Iceland ; for a coaft of 1800 miles is not eafily guarded, even if an armed veffel was kept on purpofe, efpecially as the people are the beft part of the fummer

* Mr. Anderfon fays, their weights and meafures are in general according to the ftandard of Hamburg, and that the Hamburghers were the firft that eftablifhed trade among them.

† The fame Author fays, the cunning Dutch know how to catch at an opportunity of fneaking in, the lord of the manor having no armed veffels to defend the trade, and merchant fhips, no time to lie out and watch them.

twenty

twenty or thirty miles out at fea a fifhing.   No doubt, if the
company's fhips had a commiffion given them, they would be
the beft guards of the coafts, as they fail all about the ifland.

C H A P. CII.

Concerning their religion.

WHEN the roman catholic religion took place throughout Europe, it was likewife the eftablifhed religion of this
ifland, and was not extirpated without fome effufion of blood,
occafioned chiefly by the obftinacy of a powerful and bigotted
roman catholic bifhop and his party, which however coft him his
head *.   Since the reformation, the evangelic lutheran religion,
is the only tolerated here ; notwithftanding, fome fuperftitious
notions are ftill rooted in the illiterate people, as in almoft all
other countries, though thefe fuperftitions are not properly the
refult of religious principles.

C H A P. CIII.

Concerning the ecclefiaftical ftate of this ifland.

ICELAND is divided into two bifhopricks, the eaft, fouth,
and weft quarters being allotted to one, namely, the fee of
Skalholt, and the north quarter alone, conftituting the fee of
Hoolum.   Each of thefe bifhopricks has a latin fchool, with a
rector and other affiftants under him, who teach theology, and
other branches of literature, and fit out thofe, who exhibit
proofs of their capacity, for the miniftry, and have them or-
dained priefts without going out of the ifland, or to the univerfity at Copenhagen.   Some notwithftanding repair every year
to Denmark, in order to purfue their ftudies in law or divi-
nity, at the univerfity of Copenhagen, and they generally have
the preference of thofe that have not been abroad, and get the
beft livings, and moft lucrative civil employments.   The print-

---

* Mr. Anderfon fays, the lutheran religion is the only adhered to there, except
by fome few who defcend from catholic anceftors, and ftill perfift in, and fecretly
practife fome fuperftitions.   Our author tells us, that all are defcended from catholic
anceftors, and were as ftrict catholics before the reformation, as now they are lu-
therans.

ing-

ing-office at Hoolum, once removed to Skalholt, was brought back, and is now in a very good condition. It was the legacy of one of the bifhops of Hoolum, and in it are printed religious books, and all the king's public orders, in the language of the country. In the time of the reformation, a great part of the church revenues were fecularifed, and now belong to the king. The income of each bifhoprick may amount to two thoufand rixdollars, out of which the incumbent muft keep the rector and corrector, the minifter of the cathedral church, who is the bifhop's curate to preach for him, and a certain number of fcholars, who have lodging, board, and cloathing allowed them; the cathedral and palace are likewife to be kept in repair; fo that the balance, after thefe deductions, reverting to the bifhop, cannot well amount to more than twelve hundred rixdollars per annum *. Each man pays the king a certain annual tax, called Gieftold, which amounts to about ten fifh a year. Part of this tax has been gracioufly granted by his majefty to the bifhoprick; but it is neither a bifhop's-toll, nor does the bifhop receive it of every farmer in the country; for in many places the king keeps it entire, and in others, it is farmed out to the fyffelmen, or lords of the manor. The clergy's revenues are not eafily afcertained, becaufe they do not confift in ready money, but rather in lands belonging to the refpective livings. Certain dues however, accrue to them from each farm, befides fome fees for performing certain offices. Some livings are tolerably good, fome middling, and fome very poor. To make them better for the poorer clergy, the king has given up fome of his eftates in the bifhoprick of Skalholt, and in the bifhoprick of Hoolum, allows a hundred rixdollars *per annum*, to be divided among them †. Some livings are worth two hundred rixdollars *per annum*, and the very pooreft of the clergy enjoy at leaft of the king's bounty, four

* Mr. Anderfon fays, there is a printing-houfe at each bifhop's feat, where they print religious books in the native language. He alfo fays, that the neat revenues of each bifhoprick, are only about 1200 rixdollars *per ann.*

† According to the fame Author, there is a bifhop's toll (as he calls it) which obliges every man to deliver ten fifh *per ann.* to the bifhop, and the beft livings, purfuant to his calculation, are not worth upwards of a hundred rixdollars *per ann.* and fome are fo very poor, that they do not bring in even four rixdollars a year; yet, adds he, the incumbents are not to be pitied, becaufe they behave themfelves no better than the meaneft farmer or boor.

rixdollars

rixdollars paid them every year. The clergy have neither the
tenths of fish, nor of any thing else, yet some small dues must
be paid them either in goods or money. In the Weſtman iſlands
it is cuſtomary to give the clergy a kind of tithe of each boat,
when they return from fiſhing; but this is peculiar to theſe
iſlands *. Undoubtedly, there are many poor livings in the iſland,
whereof the revenues are so ſmall, that they cannot ſupport their
reſpective miniſters, ſome of whom are obliged to have recourſe
to manual labour for maintaining their families, or to go a fiſhing
like the common people. However, their congregations are far
from being neglected, and they herein follow the example of the
apoſtle Paul, who, though he earned his bread by the labour of
his hands, was a great and edifying preacher.

C H A P. CIV.

Concerning their churches.

MOST of the churches have lands and revenues annexed
to them, as in ancient times, and ſome of later date, a
ſufficiency to ſupport them. The churches are built in the ſame
manner as their houſes, though ſomething larger, the founda-
tions being laid even with the ground, or a little higher, and the
roof covered with turf, and the inſide wainſcotted †. Theſe
churches are built proportionable to the congregations; for the
houſes and farms, as before related, being ſcattered about, there
are ſometimes only ſeven, eight or ten farms to a pariſh, though
ſome contain from ten to thirty: add to which, that as all perſons cannot appear together at church, the congregation muſt of
conſequence be in ſome churches very ſmall. The building of
their houſes and churches low, is chiefly occaſioned by the ſcarcity
of timber and bricks, of which laſt, though there is a ſufficiency
of materials to make them, yet the proceſs cannot be executed

---

* Mr. Anderſon ſays, that ſome of the clergy have part of the tithes the farmer
is obliged to pay, and ſome two thirds thereof. In other parts they have two lots
out of each boat, which are equal to two fiſhermens portion.

† The ſame Author ſays, the churches are like the farmers huts, ſunk down in the
ground, the walls of broken ſtones faſtened with twigs, clay, mortar, &c. and covered
with turf, and not larger than a common room, and ſo low, that any one may touch
the ceiling.

for

for want of fewel *. The cathedral church at Hoolum is built of frame-work, ninety-eight foot long, thirty wide, and about thirty-fix or forty high. It ftands a little higher than the ground, has a wooden fpire, and round the choir is a fine ftone wall, which was built upwards of four hundred years ago by a bifhop, who intended to finifh the whole cathedral in that manner, but died before it was completed. The frame-work of the bifhop's palace at Hoolum is of oak, and walled between. The roof is covered with boards, and no part, either top or fides, with earth, or mould. The frame-work of this houfe was made at Copenhagen, and put up and walled by bifhop Gudbrander, in 1576, as appears by the date of the year carved on the timber; fo that it now has ftood unmoved almoft two hundred years, though the foundation begins to want repair. The cathedral at Skalholt, is much the fame as that at Hoolum, except that the wall round the choir is fomething lefs. The fpire is alfo of wood, and has a bell. This church, which was built time out of mind, ftands on an eminence, and being viewed at a diftance, makes a fine appearance. The church at the king's palace of Beffefted, alfo framed and walled, and the fides and top boarded over, is about fifty foot long, twenty-five foot wide, and pretty high. The manfion-houfe is built in the fame manner, and the apartments are full nine foot high, and the walls boarded over, except the fouth-weft fide, where I obferved, that though more rain beats on that fide, than other parts, and though it had not been repaired for a great while, yet the cementing or junctures of the bricks were very clofe and tight. An old houfe two ftories high, where the king's fteward formerly lived, and where he ftill has his compting-houfe on the upper floor, has ftood fince the year 1680, though now very much decayed, and fit to be pulled down. It withftood a very great ftorm, one of the winters I was there, and I was greatly furprized that it did not then tumble down. Several other churches may be met with, which are high, and wainfcotted both within and without, and

* Mr. Anderfon fays, they are under a neceffity of building low on account of the heavy ftorms and winds that continually rage in this ifland. He alfo fays, that the Danes attempted to build a church of the ufual height in Denmark, but that the following winter, being blown down in a ftorm, they were obliged to build themfelves a low one in its ftead.

have

have been built for fome years. A handfome building in the Danifh ftile, the dwelling-place of a worthy and very confiderable man, now ftands at Thingöre cloyfter, in the parifh of Hunnevatn. In moft of the churches are altar-pieces, and fome very handfome, imported from Copenhagen. The altar is generally placed as in Denmark and moft places at the eaft end of the church, and under the altar are locked up the various ornaments, utenfils and inftruments belonging to the church. Every church has a font, which in many places is handfomely railed in like the choir: there is alfo a pew for the confeffion, in which the minifter fits till he mounts the pulpit. This pulpit ufually fo placed, that it may be feen all over the church, is conftructed and contrived after the manner of moft country places in Denmark, and in fome parts it is handfomely painted and carved. Moft churches have pews, at leaft on the women's fide, and fome have a metal fconce, or a fhip, or fome other ornament hanging up. In fhort, all the churches are exactly as I have here defcribed them, and fuch is their appearance within at all times, whether in the time of divine fervice or not. As to the ornaments, veffels and utenfils, which are only ufed during divine fervice, they are as neat and as handfome as in the country churches in Denmark. The veftments ufed by the minifter in fome churches, are made of velvet, or of rich filk, and ornamented with a crofs of gold or filver. Some have two fuits of veftments, a common, and a very elegant one for feftivals. Moft churches are in poffeffion of a cup or chalice of filver, and in fome they are gilt ; but fuch congregations as are very poor, are obliged to content themfelves with chalices of pewter. The furplices and altar cloths are of fine linen, laced or worked round, and fome churches have filk altar cloths, laced with gold and filver. A pair of large metal candlefticks generally ftand on all the altars, and a handfome piece of painting is placed over the altar, and frequently fome paintings grace the choir. In the cathedral are feveral curious pieces of antiquity, and a great many veffels and ornaments preferved fince the catholic times. The churches moft commonly belong to fome private perfons, and make part of their eftates, and as they generally refide near them, they fometimes lay up fome of their

chefts

chefts and goods in the church, or in the loft over the place of worfhip, for greater fecurity; but they never put any thing in to crowd or fill up the church *. Thefe chefts and fuch things, may alfo ferve the people to fit on, wherever benches are wanting.

CHAP. CV.

Concerning the clergy.

THOUGH feveral clergymen of this country have taken their degrees at the univerfity of Copenhagen, and have gone through their examinations with honour and great enco-miums on their merit, I will not alledge them as a proof or ar-gument, that there are good and learned divines in Iceland, be-ing willing to reftrain the matter to thofe only who were never out of the country, and who received their entire education at the king's fchools. Among thefe, is that learned and eminent divine the prefent bifhop of Skalholt, whom his Majefty thought worthy of that high employment in the church, though he did not ftudy at Co-penhagen. Befides being profoundly verfed in theology, he has gone through all the latin poets and authors, at which I was greatly furprized; but it is not to be fuppofed, that all of them are fo learned; for the old latin proverb, *ex quolibet ligno non fit mercurius*, may hold good among them, as it alfo does among us, and all other nations †. The generality of the clergy under-ftand latin and theology very well, and I myfelf have feen fome exercifes very ingenioufly executed by thofe defigned for clergy-men. I am told, they are obliged to this duty every year, be-fore the vicar and two other minifters, or the bifhop, if they live not at too great a diftance. It is fome theological theme which they are to make a differtation upon in latin, and which generally they perform admirably well. This ferves to fhew how

* Mr. Anderfon fays, that thofe who have the care of churches, are allowed for their trouble to fill them with all forts of lumber, upon which the people fit during divine fervice, there being no pews, nor any thing to fhew the appearance of a church.

† The fame Author fays, that the clergy in general are of little worth; that the greater part of them have learnt nothing; that they feldom have been any farther than the bifhop's fchools; that they can hardly read latin, and that befides, they are fad de-bauched wretches, addicted to the drinking of brandy, and getting drunk without any fhame or regard to their profeffion.

the

the clergy muſt be qualified, ſuch being even required of the young ecclefiaſtics, who muſt thereby be thought to have made no ſlender progreſs at the ſchools in Iceland. The clergy's conduct is very narrowly inſpected into, as well as that of the people in general, in regard to religious matters, and the leaſt fault is not ſuffered to go unpuniſhed. If a miniſter on a funday or holyday, ſets out only on a ſmall journey, he is immediately ſummoned to appear before a court held on purpoſe to examine into ſuch matters. I only mention this, that a judgment may be formed of the confequences of any greater miſdemeanour, for which they are either preſently ſuſpended, or ſeverely reprimand-ed. For the crime of drunkenneſs, or any other indecency, they loſe their livings, and have their gowns ſtript off *.

C H A P. CVI.

Concerning the education of their children.

THERE are no ſchools for young children, neither can any well be, the houſes, as I before obſerved, being ſcat-tered at ſuch a diſtance from one another, that it is impoſſible to bring them together in one ſchool †. The parents, and ſuch of the family as are qualified, inſtruct the young children in read-ing the articles of their religion: the miniſters alſo in viſiting their pariſhioners, frequently examine and prepare them with due care, againſt the time they are to be preſented to the biſhop for confirmation. They are kept always at home while they are young, and ſee no other examples than their parents ſet them, which are not vicious. Their diſpoſitions are mild and tender, and though not generally ſo briſk, yet they ſhew a decent kind of vivacity, eſpecially thoſe that are ſent to Copenhagen. The ſame regulations and orders that obtain in Denmark for the in-

* Mr. Anderſon ſays, that the clergyman often gets into the pulpit ſo drunk, that not able to ſtand, he is obliged to go down again, and have his place ſupplied by the clerk, who reads a ſermon to the congregation. It often happens, he adds, that the parſon, clerk and congregation, being in the ſame condition, they all leave the church without hearing or performing any worſhip at all; for ſuch bad examples muſt be at-tended with as bad conſequences.

† The ſame Author ſays, the youth are kept but a ſhort time at ſchool; for the parents rather chooſe to keep them at home, to be employed in houſhold buſineſs and other work, where to their great misfortune, they are ſeduced to all wickedneſs, by the wild and profligate examples they have before their eyes.

ſtructing

ftructing children in religion, and giving them the means of fal-
vation, by confirming them, and bringing them to the facrament,
are alfo adopted in Iceland. The excellent catechifm of that
eminent divine, bifhop Pontoppidan, is tranflated into the Iceland
language, and is ufed both in churches and private houfes.
The minifters inftruct and examine the children, and none are
admitted to the facrament of the Lord's-fupper, till they
thoroughly underftand what they are going to do; confequently, none are admitted very young, and not till their underftand-
ings ripen with their age, as it happens to young people in other
countries. I before obferved, that as they are not put very
young to labour, many of them muft be ftrong enough and able
to go a fifhing fome years before their underftanding has been
ripe enough to fit them for the Lord's-table: from whence it
may be concluded, that they are not fuffered to go very young,
and that great care is taken to have them duly prepared *.

C H A P. CVII.

Concerning the vices of the Icelanders.

THESE people have been reprefented by fome travellers as
profligate, debauched, and wicked, and in no refpect
better than favages †. In the courfe of this treatife, I have
given

---

* Mr. Anderfon fays, that on account of the danger they are expofed to at fea,
they take their children to the facrament of the Lord's-fupper at eight or nine years
of age, whence how well they are inftructed and prepared, may be eafily imagined.

† The fame Author fays, that this people know very little of God, or his will;
that they are addicted to fuperftitious practices; that for the value of two marks, or
fixteen pence, they will perjure themfelves even to the prejudice of their neareft relations, and that they are quarrelfome, full of wrath and revenge, extremely lafcivious
and vicious, and errant thieves and cheats. What then, fays he, can be expected
from a people that have no inward awe or check, and live in an unbridled licentioufnefs,
without any reftraint afhore and at fea, frequent opportunities unobferved, and confequently unpunifhable, and continually indulging themfelves in the filthy fin of drunken-
nefs? I fhall not affign, adds he, any political reafon why the magiftrates wink at
thefe enormities; and as it is not my bufinefs to criticife thereon, fhall now only mention what happened not many years ago, when this people was vifited by a fatal and
infectious fmall-pox, which almoft depopulated the ifland. In order to recruit again,
(for the people of the reft of his Danifh Majefty's dominions, had no great inclination to go there) all the young women were fuffered to have fix baftards, without
any difparagement to their character as maidens; but as thefe good natured creatures were too lavifh of their favours, the government was obliged to lay a reftraint
upon their fury, and if I may believe it, laid a punifhment upon the crime of the

N n   fame

given a very faithful and particular account of every thing relating to them, as I really found the matter, and I hope that I have convinced the world, that they are not guilty of the vices they indiscriminately stand charged with. The many that go from hence to Denmark, to learn trades, or enter into service, proves them to be a people soberly inclined, and of virtuous and good principles, their conduct being generally such, as gains them both love and esteem. They are brought up in the christian religion, which is early implanted in them: they have a conscience as well as the rest of mankind, and are not without feeling some inward reluctancy to vice: they have also magistrates, and a civil power, under whose awe they stand, to restrain and curb them, and they cannot commit an unlawful act with impunity.

C H A P. CVIII.

Concerning their nuptial ceremonies.

MARRIAGES here, as in other countries, are not always agreeable to the inclinations of the parties, but are often contracted for the sake of interest; so that it is not strange if a father or nearest relation, for very trifling reasons, refuses consent to a match; consent being here required with as much formality as in other countries. It is customary for the minister to go and ask the bride in marriage of her parents, or those that stand in their stead; after which, not many ceremonies are used at the weddings, neither have they many guests, their houses being but small *. The bride and bridegroom are attended to church by their nearest relations, and there joined in holy

---

fame nature with it, which I do not choose to explain. Our author says, this disease raged in 1707, and as out of many thousands still living, none could give him an account of any such thing, he hopes that no body will be so uncharitable as to believe it ever was so.

* Mr. Anderson says, they marry according to their inclinations and circumstances, with very few ceremonies, and are attended to the church by their nearest relations on both sides, where they are joined by the parson. Afterwards the bride, bridegroom and parson, placing themselves against one of the walls, with the relations on each side of them, a cup of brandy is given to the bride, who drinks to her next neighbour, and by way of setting a good example, drinks it all up: the bridegroom on his side does the same, and thus the cups of brandy go round, till they can neither hold them, nor stand on their legs.

wedlock

wedlock by the minister, which is generally performed on a sunday before the minister goes into the pulpit. When the sermon and service are over, they repair to the house where the bride came from, and have an entertainment according to their circumstances, and drink and rejoice with moderation and decency. As it is usual with them on such occasions to regale themselves with a little brandy, it accordingly goes round; but they have neither music nor dancing, and when the feast is over, all retire to their respective habitations.

C H A P. CIX.

Whether the Icelanders are fond of the game of chess.

IT cannot be alledged as matter of fact, that the Icelanders are lovers of gaming. It is true, they divert themselves a little at chess, as also at cards, but in a more particular manner at the former, in which they are very expert, though not such great masters of it, as in all probability their forefathers were [*]. Their chief leisure time they have is in the fishing seasons, when the weather is so bad that they cannot venture out to sea, and then it is that a great many being mustered together from the north and east, make parties to divert themselves, and pass away the time [†]. In the winter long evenings, they have employment enough in their families.

C H A P. CX.

Concerning their manner of dancing.

THEY have no idea of dancing, though sometimes the merchants at the factories for their diversion will get a fiddle and make them dance, in which they succeed no better than by hopping and jumping about [‡]. When they have been

[*] Mr. Anderson says, that they apply themselves very much to the game of chess, and are as well as their ancestors, very eminent in, and great masters of it.

[†] The same Author says, they have a deal of leisure time upon their hands, when the fishing season is over, and during the long nights; and as they do not choose to do more work than they cannot help, they usually go to chess.

[‡] He also says, that they are very fond of dancing, which they perform with many antics, the men and women standing facing each other, and so jigging it from one foot to the other.

treated

treated and made merry, they generally fall a finging, and have great variety of heroic fongs, which as having no fkill in mufical modulations, they roar out in a very harfh and uncouth manner.

C H A P. CXI.

Concerning their civil government.

THE Icelanders have a ftiftf-amptmand or governor, and an amptmand or deputy-governor. The former is generally chofen out of the nobility, as Güldenlove, Güldencrone, and the prefent count Rantzou, who is alfo one of the lords of the bed-chamber to his majefty *. Such generally refide in Copenhagen, but the amptmand or deputy governor, always refides in Iceland, at the king's palace of Beffefted, and is fometimes a nobleman. His falary is four hundred rixdollars in crowns *per annum*. Befides the deputy-governor, the king has a receiver or land-fteward, who collects throughout the ifland all taxes and revenues, and fends in his accounts to the king's exchequer. This receiver or fteward, had hitherto always lived at Beffefted, with the deputy-governor, but has now the liberty to refide at the abbey of Widöe. The king allowed him a falary of three hundred and fifty rixdollars *per ann.* in crowns, but lately made an addition thereto of a hundred.

C H A P. CXII.

Concerning the reft of his majefty's fervants or officers in the ifland.

BESIDES the above officers, there are perfons called fyffelmen over certain diftricts, who farm the king's taxes, and account with his land-fteward for what they have agreed. By this means they acquire a handfome livelihood †. The land-fteward is always fyffelman or tax-gatherer himfelf in the diftrict

---

* Mr. Anderfon fays, that the amptmand or deputy-governor, is not of the nobility, but generally one who has been a fecretary, or a well deferving domeftic to fome minifter of ftate at court, who has obtained from the king this confiderable employment for him, as a reward for his faithful fervices.

† The fame Author fays, that the deputy-governor has a falary of four hundred rixdollars fpecie, befides perquifites or fees, which amount to as much again, and that he is the fupreme judge in civil and criminal affairs. The receiver or land-fteward has, he fays, two hundred rixdollars *per ann.* falary.

of Guldbringe, where he refides, and as he has a ftanding falary as land-fteward, he muft account with the rent-chamber or exchequer, for the taxes and other dues in this diftrict. The reft of the king's revenues arife from the company, who pay an annual fum to the king in the rent-chamber or exchequer of this ifland. The revenues of the fecularifed abbey-lands, and other lands belonging to the king which are farmed out, are paid to the fteward *. The amount of thefe accounts is not eafily afcertained, as not being every year alike. As to judges, there are two, called laugmænd; the one has the fouth and eaft department, the other the north and weft, and fometimes one or two deputies are allowed them. The ifland contains eighteen diftricts or fyffeler, and each has a fyffelman or tax-gatherer, but Mule and Skaftefield to the eaft have two each: there is alfo one in the Weftman-iflands, fo that the whole number throughout the country amounts to twenty-one. One of the tax-gatherers or fyffelmen in Mule diftrict, who fuperintends the fouth and middle divifion, has fifteen courts to attend at certain times of the year, and in the beginning of the year, when the court is held at Mandtal, has a journey of three hundred Englifh miles to make. This I only mention to fhew, what a confiderable diftrict fome have under them. Thefe fyffelmen act as juftices of the peace, each in his diftrict, and are like a kind of deputy-ftewards, or what they call Herredsfogder in Denmark †. As they have a genteel income, and are generally people of property, they are very much refpected in the ifland.

* Mr. Anderfon fays, that the harbours are farmed out to the company for twenty thoufand fpecie dollars; that the feveral eftates of the king bring in eight thoufand dollars more; that in fome diftricts he has one third of the tithes of the fifh, and that each fubject who is worth more than twenty dollars, muft give him forty fifh a year; our author has before obferved, that there is no tithe of fifh paid here to the clergy.

† The fame author fays, there are three laugmænd, in Danifh, Lands-dommere, that is, judges, who have each a particular diftrict, and twenty-four fyffelmen or taxgatherers, each alfo having a village or fmall diftrict under him, like the herredsfogder in Denmark.

CHAP.

C H A P. CXIII.

Concerning their laws.

ALL suits in law concerning inheritance and property, and every thing relating to *meum* and *tuum*, are decided by the old Iceland law; but with regard to freehold property, the Norwegian law takes place. The old ecclesiastical law is entirely abolished, and is only referred to in case of tithes, all other spiritual matters being decided by the second book of the Norwegian law, or by royal edicts. In the year 1564, the two laugmænd or judges then living, in conjunction with twenty-four other men elected for that purpose, made a law relating to pawns and forfeitures, which was confirmed and put in force the year following, by order of king Frederic the second, and dated from Lund the 13th of April 1565 *. Pursuant to the tenour of that law, all forfeits and pawns are to this day adjudged, and brought to a final determination : it is very concise, the whole being comprised in two pages. Crimes and misdemeanours are canvassed according to the first and sixth book of the Norwegian laws of king Christian V. besides which, several royal edicts and orders must be consulted. His late majesty king Frederic IV. having ordered some of the most able lawyers to compose a new book of laws for Iceland, it was accordingly executed, and now only waits for his present majesty's approbation and royal authority. There is more work for lawyers here than one would imagine, especially in (Odels-sager) or cases relative to freehold and trespasses, the inhabitants suing each other at law upon the least encroachment on their respective grounds, or with regard to things, in which they presume their property is invalidated. So obstinate are they, though they have grounds of some Danish miles extent lying between them, that one will

---

* Mr. Anderson says, that all civil matters relating chiefly to inheritance, or hereditary right, are decided by the ancient Iceland law-book, which was made by king Magnus, surnamed Lagabætter, or rectifier of the laws. Spiritual affairs are judged by the christnaret, or *jus ecclesiasticum*, and the great book of judgment established by king Frederic the second; and misdemeanors, by a book of laws made by king Christian the fifth. His late majesty king Frederic the fourth, had ordered some learned persons in the law, to prepare a new code for Iceland, which now has lain some years in Denmark for his majesty's approbation.

not

not permit the other to enjoy the least spot without his making some return for it, though in the main, of no use to himself*. Sometimes suits of some importance happen; but I have seen actions brought against people, and carried into the upper courts, though the whole contest regarded perhaps not the value of a dollar, and this by the perverse selfishness of the richer sort. Their manner of proceeding at law is as follows. In the first place, after the action is brought, they are to appear at a court within the district where the offence has happened. The sysselman of the district presides in this court as justice, and passes sentence. From hence they appeal to the langret, which is held at Oxeraae, and begins every year the eighth of July, and lasts as long as there is any business to do. Each laugmænd or judge, decrees alone in his own department, and has eight laugrettemænd or assessors on the bench with him. From this court an appeal may be lodged at the highest in the island, which is held at the same time, and in which the amptmand or deputy-governor presides, who has for assessors the judge, whose sentence or decree has not been given in this cause before, and as many sysselmen, or in default of them, laugrættemænd, as make twelve exclusive of the deputy-governor, who is president, or in his absence, the king's land-steward. This court in respect to the forms, is like the (ober hoff-ret) or the highest court in Norway, wherein an inferior judge for prevaricating, or declining to do justice may be indicted. From this court there is an appeal to the superior court at Copenhagen, provided the cause is of such consequence as is set forth in the Norwegian law. In spiritual cases, the dean has a court, which consists of himself and two assessors, and from it an appeal may be lodged in the consistorial court, which is held also at Oxeraae, for the diocese of Skalholt, the same time the other court is fitting. The amptmand or deputy-governor presides here, and the bishops, deans and clergy, are assessors. This same court for the diocese of Hoolum, is held after Michaelmas, at a place called Flyge Myre, about three Danish miles from Hoolum, and to it the governor generally deputes

* Mr. Anderson says, that in all probability there cannot be many law-suits in Iceland between the inhabitants, though in former times, disputes frequently arose between the bishops and the king's stewards, which were seldom decided but by an appeal to the king.

some

fome perfon in his room.   From this court there is alfo an appeal to the fuperior court at Copenhagen.   No proctors are appointed in Iceland, though in each caufe the deputy-governor
may conftitute fuch as he thinks proper.

CHAP. CXIV.

Concerning executions, or punifhments by death.

NO other ways are ufed to punifh by death than beheading
with an ax, or hanging.   The women are thruft into a
fack and drowned.   The fyffelman does not perform this office,
but keeps at his own expence a perfon for this purpofe *.

CHAP. CXV.

Conclufion.

BY living in Iceland upwards of two years, I had an opportunity of feeing a great part of the country, and detecting
the groundlefs affertions, and falfe afperfions of fuch travellers
as endeavoured to depreciate this ifland.   I have faid nothing
but what may be deemed a genuine picture of it, reprefented in
true and faithful colours, chiefly for the inftruction and amufe-
ment of thofe who may be defirous to conceive a juft idea of
Iceland.

* Mr. Anderfon fays, that the inferior judge or fyffelman, executes the law both
in criminal and civil cafes, which our Author denies, and fays, they keep execu-
tioners on purpofe.   He adds, that when a malefactor is hanged, they keep him in
agony a good while before he can give up the ghoft.

METEORO-

METEOROLOGICAL

OBSERVATIONS

MADE AT

BESSESTED in ICELAND,

From Auguſt 1, 1749, to July 31, 1751.

P p

Auguſt	1	Clear and fine weather.
Saturday	2	Clear and cloudy by turns with ſome wind.
Sunday	3	Clear and fine weather, with very little wind.
Monday	4	Forenoon clear weather, towards noon a little rain.
Tueſday	5	Cloudy by intervals, and the wind ſomewhat high.
Wedneſday	6	Cloudy with a little wind.
Thurſday	7	Calm and fine weather.
Friday	8	Clear and calm weather.
Saturday	9	Calm weather, but ſomewhat cloudy.
Sunday	10	Clear and calm weather.
Monday	11	Fine weather with a little wind.
Tueſday	12	Clear weather and windy.
Wedneſday	13	Calm weather and cloudy.
Thurſday	14	Clear and calm weather.
Friday	15	Cloudy with ſome wind, but towards evening the wind very high.
Saturday	16	Cloudy, with very little wind.
Sunday	17	Clear weather and a little wind.
Monday	18	Cloudy and ſomewhat windy.
Tueſday	19	Clear weather and pretty windy.
Wedneſday	20	Heavy cloudy weather, with a very high wind.
Thurſday	21	Stormy weather, which continued during the whole night.
Friday	22	Rainy weather, with a little wind.
Saturday	23	Calm and ſtill.
Sunday	24	Clear weather, with a high wind.
Monday	25	Rainy weather, and ſomewhat windy.
Tueſday	26	The ſame, but the wind not ſo high.
Wedneſday	27	Rainy, but calm.
Thurſday	28	Calm with clouds in the morning and forenoon, but the wind high in the afternoon.
Friday	29	Clear and calm weather.
Saturday	30	Calm, but dark weather.
Sunday	31	Rainy, with bluſtring winds.
September	1	The wind very high, and ſometimes accompanied by rain.
Tueſday	2	Clear for the greater part of the day, and pretty windy.

		Wind.	Barom.	Ther.	
Auguſt		1. N. W.	27 11-	11-	ſupra degel.
Saturday		2. S. E.	28 0	12	
Sunday		3. N. E.	28 0	12-	
Monday		4. S. E. 12 cl. N.	27 9-	13	
Tuefday		5. N.	27 9	13	
Wednefday		6. S. by E.	27 9-	12	
Thurfday		7. N. E.	27 10	12-	
Friday		8. N.	27 9-	13	
Saturday		9. N.	27 9 0	12	
Sunday		10. N.	27 11	13	
Monday		11. N.	28 1-	12	
Tuefday		12. N.	27 10	12	
Wednefday		13. W. S. W.	27 10 0	11	
Thurfday		14. N.	27 11-	11 0	
Friday		15. N.	27 9	11	
		N. by E.	27 7		
Saturday		16. N. by E.	27 7 0	11	
Sunday		17. N.	27 7-	10-	
Monday		18. N. to E.	27 6-	11-	
Tuefday		19. N. E.	27 4-	11-	
Wednefday		20. N. E.	27 4-	9	
Thurfday		21. N. E.	27 8	7	
Friday		22. N. W.	27 10	8-	
Saturday		23. E. to N.	27 7	9-	
Sunday		24. N. E.	27 8 0	8	
Monday		25. S.	28 1 0	10-	
Tuefday		26. S. W.	27 10 0	10-	
Wednefday		27. S	27 7-	11-	
Thurfday		28. N.	27 5	11-	
Friday		29. N. N. E.	27 7	11	North light.
Saturday		30. S.	27 10 0	10	
Sunday		31. S.	27 9	10-	
September		1. S.	27 8	9-	
Tuefday		2. S.	27 11-	9-	

Wednef.

1749.		The weather.
September	3	The wind very high, with fome fhowers of rain, towards the evening a great ftorm, which continued very violent all night.
Thurſday	4	Very ftormy with rain.
Friday	5	Clear and cloudy by intervals, with a little wind, but towards evening the wind very high.
Saturday	6	The weather like that of the preceding day.
Sunday	7	Calm weather; but for the better part cloudy.
Monday	8	Rainy and calm.
Tueſday	9	Very windy and cloudy, a pretty fharp froft in the night.
Wedneſday	10	Clear weather, froft and the wind fomewhat high.
Thurſday	11	Clear and calm weather.
Friday	12	Rainy and calm weather.
Saturday	13	Clear weather, and windy.
Sunday	14	Clear and calm.
Monday	15	Dark weather, and a little windy.
Tueſday	16	Calm and mild weather.
Wedneſday	17	Clear calm weather with fome froft.
Thurſday	18	Stormy weather with fome rain.
Friday	19	Rainy and windy.
Saturday	20	Dark weather with a little wind.
Sunday	21	Clear, and by intervals windy.
Monday	22	Cloudy, with a little wind.
Tueſday	23	Clear, and the greater part of the day calm.
Wedneſday	24	Rainy, but calm weather.
Thurſday	25	The wind very high, with fome fhowers of rain.
Friday	26	Cloudy, and pretty windy.
Saturday	27	Clear, and for the greater part calm.
Sunday	28	Clear and calm till noon, but in the afternoon windy.
Monday	29	Rainy with fome wind, the afternoon a pretty great ftorm.
Tueſday	30	Very windy and cloudy.
October	1	For the better part clear but fomewhat windy.
Thurſday	2	The wind very high, with fome fhowers of rain.
Friday	3	Rainy and windy.
Saturday	4	Clear the greater part of the day, and fomewhat windy.

	Wind.	Barom.	Ther.	
September	3. S.	28 1 ʊ	10-	
Thursday	4. S.	27 8	10-	
Friday	5. S.	27 11-	9-	
Saturday	6. S. to W.	27 10	9	
Sunday	7. S. to E.	28 1-	9 ʊ	
Monday	8. E.	27 7	10	Strong north light.
Tuesday	9. N. E.	27 10	8 ʊ	
Wednesday	10. N.	28 3	4	
Thursday	11. E. N. E.	28 2	4-	
Friday	12. E.	27 10 ʊ	6	
Saturday	13. N. E.	27 9 ʊ	7	Strong north light.
Sunday	14. S,	27 6-	5	
Monday	15. E.	27 6-	7	
Tuesday	16. S.	27 9-	7-	
Wednesday	17. S.W.	27 11-	6	
Thursday	18. S. S. E.	27 1-	7	
Friday	19. S. E.	27 2	7	
Saturday	20. S.	26 11	8	
Sunday	21. N. E.	27 6	9	
Monday	22. S. E.	27 10	8	
Tuesday	23. S. E.	27 7	8-	
Wednes.	24. S.	27 7	8-	
Thursday	25. S. E.	27 2-	7	
Friday	26. N. E.	27 5	8 ʊ	
Saturday	27. E.	27 7-	8	
Sunday	28. N. E.	28 0-	7-	
Monday	29. S. S. E.	28 2	6 ʊ	
	S. W.	27 7		
Tuesday	30. W.	27 6 ʊ	7	
October	1. N. E.	27 6 ʊ	5	North light.
Thursday	2. S. E.	27 7 ʊ	5	
Friday	3. W. S. W.	27 9	8	North light.
Saturday	4. S. W.	28 1	6-	

Q q   October

1749.		The weather.
October	5	Some rain with brisk gales of wind.
Monday	6	Gloomy weather with a very high wind.
Tuesday	7	Rainy with a very high wind.
Wednesday	8	Rainy and very windy.
Thursday	9	Rainy and windy.
Friday	10	Clear and calm during almost the whole day.
Saturday	11	Dark weather, pretty windy, and towards noon a great storm.
Sunday	12	Changeable weather with rain and hail, clear, windy and stormy.
Monday	13	Dark weather, and pretty windy.
Tuesday	14	Fine calm weather, but in the night frost and snow.
Wednesday	15	Clear and calm weather during the better part of the day.
Thursday	16	Clear and calm with some frost.
Friday	17	Clear and calm with a slight frost.
Saturday	18	Gloomy weather, but no frost; in the afternoon and evening a great storm.
Sunday	19	Cloudy and pretty windy; a violent storm in the afternoon and night.
Monday	20	Rainy with a very high wind.
Tuesday	21	Rainy and windy.
Wednesday	22	The same.
Thursday	23	Dark weather and pretty windy.
Friday	24	For the greater part clear, with a little wind.
Saturday	25	Dark, but calm weather.
Sunday	26	Rainy and pretty windy.
Monday	27	The same.
Tuesday	28	The same.
Wednesday	29	The same; some frost in the night.
Thursday	30	Thick snow and pretty windy.
Friday	31	The same, with high winds.
November	1	Thick, hazy, cloudy, but calm; at 11 o'clock P. M. rain and snow, with a high wind.
Sunday	2	Rainy and pretty windy.
Monday	3	Clear and calm with some frost.
Tuesday	4	Clear frosty weather, with some wind.

	Wind.	Barom.		Ther.	
October	5. S.	28	2–	6–	North light.
Monday	6. S. E.	28	3	7	
Tuefday	7. S. to E.	28	3–	8	
Wednefday	8. S.	27	10	9	
Thurfday	9. S. W.	28	0 ᴜ	7–	
Friday	10. N. W.	27	11	8	North light.
Saturday	11. S. E.	28	1 ᴜ	6–	
		27	11		
	S.				
Sunday	12.	27	9	6–	
Monday	13. S.	27	6–	5 ᴜ	
Tuefday	14. W.	27	5–	4–	
Wednefday	15. S.	27	5 ᴜ	4	Strong north light.
Thurfday	16. N.		9	4	
Friday	17. S. E.		10	4	North light.
Saturday	18. E.		9–	5	
			3–		
Sunday	19. S.		8–	5–	
Monday	20. S.		8	8	
Tuefday	21. S.		10	5–	
Wednefday	22. S. E.	28	1	6–	
Thurfday	23. W.	27	10–	5	
Friday	24. W.	28	3 ᴜ	6	
Saturday	25. S.		3 ᴜ	6	
Sunday	26. E. S. E.	28	0	7	
Monday	27. S. W.	27	11	6–	
Tuefday	28. W.		8	6	
Wednefday	29. S. E.	28	1	5	Strong north light.
Thurfday	30. S. W.	27	5	4	
Friday	31. W. N. W.		6	3–	
November	1. E.		11	2–	
	S.		3	3	
Sunday	2. S.		3–	2–	
Monday	3. E.		9 ᴜ	1	North light.
Tuefday	4. N. E.		9 ᴜ	0 ᴜ	

November

1749.   The weather.

November	5	Clear frosty weather, with some wind.
Thursday	6	Clear, calm and frosty; after the north light a very high wind in the night.
Friday	7	Rainy, and a very high wind; at 11 o'clock, P.M.
Saturday	8	Dark and calm weather.
Sunday	9	Rainy with a little wind.
Monday	10	Dark and calm weather.
Tuesday	11	The same.
Wednesday	12	Snow, but calm.
Thursday	13	Clear and frosty; some wind in the afternoon, with rain and storm.
Friday	14	Rain and hail, with a very high wind.
Saturday	15	For the greater part clear and calm, with a little frost.
Sunday	16	Thick hazy weather, and somewhat windy.
Monday	17	Clear and calm weather, with a little frost.
Tuesday	18	Pretty clear and calm weather.
Wednesday	19	Clear frosty weather, and pretty windy.
Thursday	20	Rainy and windy.
Friday	21	Cloudy and very windy.
Saturday	22	Thick, but calm.
Sunday	23	Thick heavy air, and somewhat windy.
Monday	24	Rain, with a little wind.
Tuesday	25	The same.
Wednesday	26	The same, but less wind.
Thursday	27	Thick, hazy and windy.
Friday	28	The same, but somewhat milder.
Saturday	29	Calm and clear during the better part of the day.
Sunday	30	Hazy weather and pretty windy.
December	1	The same, but in the evening a storm.
Tuesday	2	Dark weather, and pretty windy.
Wednesday	3	The same, but the wind higher.
Thursday	4	The same, but less wind.
Friday	5	Thick and hazy, but for the greater part calm.
Saturday	6	Cloudy but calm, with some frost.
Sunday	7	Clear, calm, and frosty weather.
Monday	8	Rain, with some wind.
Tuesday	9	Cloudy, but calm.

	Wind.	Barom.	Ther.	
November	5. N. E.	11	1 o	infra degel.
Thurſday	6. S. E.	28 3 o	1	North light.
Friday	7. S. E.	27 8-	2-	ſupr. degel.
		3-		
Saturday	8. S.	6 o	3-.	
Sunday	9. S.	27 4	5	
Monday	10. S. E.	6-	3	
Tueſday	11. S.	4-	3-	North light.
Wedneſday	12. W.	4-	3	North light.
Thurſday	13. S. E.	7	1-	
		o-		
Friday	14. S.	2-.	3	North light.
Saturday	15. S.	4	2	North light.
Sunday	16. N. E.	5-	2	North light.
Monday	17. E. S. E.	5	2-	
Tueſday	18. E.	6 o	3 o	North light.
Wedneſday	19. N. E.	28 1	2 o	
Thurſday	20. S.	27 11-	6	
Friday	21. W.	28 1	4-	
Saturday	22. S.	7	4	
Sunday	23. S. E.	7 o	4	
Monday	24. S.	2-	5-	
Tueſday	25. S.	2	5-	
Wedneſday	26. S. E.	2	5	
Thurſday	27. S.	27 11	5-	
Friday	28. S.	28 0	6	
Saturday	29. W.	28 0	6	
Sunday	30. S.	28 2	7	
December	1. S.	28 2 o	7	
		27 8		
Tueſday	2. S. W.	28 1 o	5-	
Wedneſday	3. S. S. E.	27 11	5-	
Thurſday	4. S.	9	6-	
Friday	5. W.	4	6	North light.
Saturday	6. N. E.	27 9	2-	North light.
Sunday	7. E. S. E.	28 5	1-	North light.
Monday	8. E. S. E.	2-	2	North light.
Tueſday	9. E. S. E.	1-	4-	

1749.		The weather.

December 10 Cloudy but calm.
Thurſday 11 For the moſt part clear and calm with ſome froſt.
Friday 12 Foggy, but calm weather and a thaw.
Saturday 13 Thick weather and pretty windy.
Sunday 14 Clouds driving and wafted by ſome wind.
Monday 15 Clear and calm with froſt.
Tueſday 16 The ſame, but ſome ſnow.
Wedneſday 17 Cloudy, with ſome wind and froſt.
Thurſday 18 Hazy weather and very windy ; in the afternoon and night a ſtorm.
Friday 19 For the better part clear and pretty windy.
Saturday 20 Clear weather, ſomewhat ſtormy by guſts, and in the night a conſiderable ſtorm.
Sunday 21 Cloudy and ſtormy weather.
Monday 22 Clear and calm froſty weather, but about 2 o'clock, P. M. ſtormy with hail and ſnow.
Tueſday 23 Clear and calm weather, during almoſt the whole day. The ſame day I obſerved an eclipſe of the moon, which was total, and began almoſt at 6 o'clock, P. M. and ended 20 minutes after 8. The ſame time a beautiful north light was ſeen with two bright bows in the north, and with bright flaming rays at W. N. W. and E. N. E.
Wedneſday 24 Foggy weather and pretty windy.
Thurſday 25 Clear weather and very windy.
Friday 26 Clear, calm and mild weather.
Saturday 27 The ſame.
Sunday 28 The ſame.
Monday 29 Thick weather and pretty windy.
Tueſday 30 Rain and very high winds.
Wedneſday 31 Mild and calm weather with clouds.
1750.
January 1 Gloomy but calm weather ; in the night ſtormy.
Friday 2 Very high winds and cloudy.
Saturday 3 Stormy with rain and hail.
Sunday 4 The ſame.
Monday 5 Clouds driving, and pretty windy.

	Wind.	Barom.	Ther.	
December	10. S.	1 ᴜ	3-	
Thurſday	11. N. E. &S.E.	2	3	North light.
Friday	12. S. E. & S.	2	3-	
Saturday	13. S. & S. W.	27 9-	6-	
Sunday	14. W.	7-	4-	North light.
Monday	15. N.	8-	2-	
Tueſday	16. W. N. W.	8-	2 ᴜ	North light.
Wedneſday	17. E.	10 ᴜ	3	infra degel.
Thurſday	18. N. E.	6 ᴜ	2	North light.
Friday	19. N. E.	10 ᴜ	3-	
Saturday	20. N. E.	10	2-	
Sunday	21. N. E.	28 0	4-	
Monday	22. S. E.	1	3-	North light.
Tueſday	23. S.	27 10 / 6 ᴜ	0	
Wedneſday	24. N.	27 4 ᴜ	2	ſupr. degel.
Thurſday	25. N.	10-	1-	North light.
Friday	26. S.	28 4 ᴜ	2	infra degel.
Saturday	27. S.	4	3-	North light.
Sunday	28. S.	4-	4	
Monday	29. S. E.	2-	1-	North light.
Tueſday	30. S. E.	27 8 ᴜ	3	ſupr. degel.
Wedneſday	31. S. E.	10	3-	North light.
1750.				
January	1. E. S. E.	27 10-	3⸗	ſupr. degel.
Friday	2. S.	6	5	
Saturday	3. S.	8-	6-	
Sunday	4. S.	11	6-	
Monday	5. S.	28 ₹ ᴜ	5	

January

January	6	Cloudy but mild.
Wednefday	7	Clear and mild weather.
Thurfday	8	Cloudy but pretty windy.
Friday	9	Cloudy mild and calm ; towards midnight a storm, which ceafed by day-break.
Saturday	10	Cloudy and a little windy.
Sunday	11	Very high wind with rain about 1 o'clock, P.M.
Monday	12	By intervals cloudy and pretty windy.
Tuefday	13	Clear weather with fome wind.
Wednefday	14	Some fnow, and a little wind.
Thurfday	15	Very windy between whiles, with hail and fnow.
Friday	16	Pretty windy with fnow.
Saturday	17	Very high wind and rain.
Sunday	18	Snowy and pretty windy.
Monday	19	Windy and a thick fog with fnow.
Tuefday	20	Clear and gentle weather, with a little fnow and wind.
Wednefday	21	Calm weather, and by intervals fnow.
Thurfday	22	Clear and calm.
Friday	23	The fame.
Saturday	24	Cloudy and pretty windy ; no froft.
Sunday	25	Dark weather, with very high winds.
Monday	26	Cloudy and pretty windy.
Tuefday	27	The fame.
Wednefday	28	Clouds driving, with a high wind and fnow in the night.
Thurfday	29	Between whiles clear, with little wind.
Friday	30	Cloudy and pretty windy.
Saturday	31	Rain and very high wind; in the evening and night a ftorm.
February	1	The fame, ceafed at noon, and was fucceeded by fnow.
Monday	2	A ftorm, which was allayed in the afternoon by rain.
Tuefday	3	Hazy, with fnow and wind.
Wednefday	4	The fame.
Thurfday	5	High winds, with fnow hail and rain.
Friday	6	Clear and calm weather with a gentle froft.

	Wind.	Barom.	Ther.	
January	6. S.		2-	3-	North light.
Wednefday	7. S. S. E.		0	3	Strong north light.
Thurfday	8. S. E.	27	9 ʊ	3	)
Friday	9. S. E.		6 ʊ	3	
			3		
Saturday	10. S. S. E.		2	4	Strong north light.
Sunday	11. S. E.	26	7~	3~	
	S.		4-		North light.
Monday	12. S.		9 ʊ	3	
Tuefday	13. S.	27	0	0-	North light.
Wednefday	14. S.		4	0	
Thurfday	15. S. W.		3-	0	
Friday	16. N. W.	26	10-	0	
Saturday	17. S. E.	27	7-	1 ʊ	
Sunday	18. S. W.		6	2	
Monday	19. S. W.		5¼	0	
Tuefday	20. S. W.		1-	0	
Wednefday	21. S. W.		3	0	
Thurfday	22. N.		6	1	infra degel.
Friday	23. E.		11	5 ʊ	North light.
Saturday	24. S. E.	28	0 ʊ	1	in open air.
Sunday	25. S.	27	6-	4	fupr. degel.
Monday	26. S. S. W.		5	6	
Tuefday	27. S. W.		1	4	
Wednefday	28. W. S. W.	27	3	3	fupr. degel. North light.
Thurfday	29. W. S. W.		5-	2	
Friday	30. W.		11	2 ʊ	
Saturday	31. S.		9	6 ʊ	
February	1. S.		4 ʊ	5-	North light.
Monday	2. S.		0	2	
Tuefday	3. S. E.		1	1	North light.
Wednefday	4. S. E.		3	2	North light.
Thurfday	5. S. E.	26	10	2	
Friday	6. S.	27	2-	2 ʊ	North light.

February

1750.   The weather.

February	7	Cloudy, with a little wind and froft.
Sunday	8	Clear and calm with fome froft.
Monday	9	Cloudy and windy.
Tuefday	10	Rain with fome wind.
Wednefday	11	Clear and calm during the greater part of the day.
Thurfday	12	Cloudy with fome wind; the afternoon clear and calm.
Friday	13	Clear and calm, with fome froft.
Saturday	14	For the moft part clear and calm.
Sunday	15	Clear and calm with fome froft; but in the evening high winds, which blew into a ftorm during the night.
Monday	16	Clear weather, but very windy.
Tuefday	17	Clear, with a little wind.
Wednefday	18	Clear and pretty windy.
Thurfday	19	Clear and calm.
Friday	20	The fame.
Saturday	21	The fame; but in the night a little fnow.
Sunday	22	Clear, with a little wind.
Monday	23	The fame; but in the night fnow.
Tuefday	24	Cloudy, with a little wind.
Wednefday	25	Hazy and windy weather with a little froft.
Thurfday	26	Clear and calm, with a little froft and high winds in the night.
Friday	27	Rain and ftorm till 11 o'clock A. M. afterwards fome rain and wind, in the night fome fnow.
Saturday	28	Snow, with a little wind; but in the afternoon clear and calm weather.
March	1	Clear and calm with froft; and in the evening fome ftorms of rain and fleet.
Monday	2	Windy, with ftorms of fleet and rain.
Tuefday	3	For the moft part clear and fomewhat windy; but in the night fnow.
Wednefday	4	Cloudy with a little wind; in the evening and night very high winds with fnow, and a froft.
Thurfday	5	Clouds driving, pretty windy, and a little fnow.

	Wind.	Barom.		Ther.	
February	7. S. W.		. 2-	1	Strong north night.
Sunday	8. W.		6-	1	Strong north light.
Monday	9. N. E.		4 °	1	North light.
Tuesday	10. E. N. E.	26	8 °	4	North light.
Wednesday	11. E.		5-	4	North light.
Thursday	12. S. W.	27	2-	3	North light.
Friday	13. E. S. E.		5	2	North light.
Saturday	14. E. S. E.		7	1	
Sunday	15. E.		5	1	Strong north light.
	N. E.				
Monday	16. N.		7	1	North light.
Tuesday	17. N.E.&S.E.		9	0	North light.
Wednesday	18. S. E.		6	1	
Thursday	19. S. W.		1-	2	
Friday	20. E.		6 °	2	North light.
Saturday	21. E.		5-	2	
Sunday	22. E.		1-	3	North light.
Monday	23. E. S. E.		2-	2	
Tuesday	24. S. S. W.		7-	2	Strong north light.
Wednesday	25. N.	27	3-	1-	fupr. degel.
Thursday	26. E. S. E.		7	0	
	S.				
Friday	27. S.		0	3	North light.
Saturday	28. E. S. E.		0	2-	
March	1. E.		6	1	
		26	11		North light.
Monday	2. S.		9-	3 °	
Tuesday	3. W. S. W.	27.	4	2-	
Wednesday	4. N.		1 °	3	North light.
		26	9 °	0	
Thursday	5. E. S. E.	27	2-	0	Strong north light.

March

March	6	Pretty clear, with some wind and frost.
Saturday	7	For the most part clear and mild weather, with some frost.
Sunday	8	Clear weather, with some wind and frost.
Monday	9	Clear weather but stormy and frosty; the afternoon cloudy, stormy and frosty.
Tuesday	10	Clear weather with high winds and frost; in the afternoon cloudy and less wind.
Wednesday	11	Hazy weather, with some wind and a mild rain.
Thursday	12	Rainy and somewhat windy.
Friday	13	Cloudy with a little wind.
Saturday	14	Dark weather, and pretty windy.
Sunday	15	Between whiles clear, cloudy and windy.
Monday	16	Clear and calm weather during almost the whole day.
Tuesday	17	Cloudy and somewhat windy with a little frost; in the evening and night the wind was very high, and accompanied by snow.
Wednesday	18	For the most part clear, the wind pretty high, and a little frost; but in the afternoon a thaw, with sleet and rain.
Thursday	19	Sudden showers of rain and storms; by intervals clear, and in the evening and night calm and mild.
Friday	20	Dark, but calm weather.
Saturday	21	Unsettled weather, wind, hail, snow, and a little frost suceeding each other.
Sunday	22	Some snow and wind, no frost; but between whiles furious and blustring storms.
Monday	23	Thaw, snow and wind.
Tuesday	24	Stormy and some rain.
Wednesday	25	Very high winds with thick snow and hard frost.
Thursday	26	The wind high with showers of snow; but by intervals clear and calm.
Friday	27	Clear weather, with some wind and frost.
Saturday	28	The forenoon clear and calm; but the afternoon snowy and frosty.
Sunday	29	Gloomy weather, with some wind and frost, and showers of snow, sleet and rain.

1750.

	Wind.	Barom.		Ther.	
March	6. S.		2-	1	Strong north light.
Saturday	7. N. N. W.		4	1	North light.
Sunday	8. E. S. E.		2-	1	infra degel.
Monday	9. N.		1	2	
			9	6-	in the open air.
Tuesday	10. N.	28	4-	7	in the open air.
	S. E.		6		
Wednesday	11. S. W.		1	1	
Thursday	12. S. W.	27	8	4	supr. degel.
Friday	13. S. W.		6	4	
Saturday	14. W. S. W.		8 ꝺ	4-	
Sunday	15. W. S. W.		8	2-	
Monday	16. N. & E.		8	2	
Tuesday	17. E.		9	1	
Wednesday	18. E.		6	1 ꝺ	
	S. E.		3	3	
Thursday	19. S.	26	10	4	
Friday	20. N. W.		10-	3	
Saturday	21. S. W.	27	1 ꝺ	1-	
Sunday	22. S. W.	27	2	2	North light. supra degel.
Monday	23. S. W.		4	2	North light.
Tuesday	24. S. W.	26	5-	4	
Wednesday	25. S. W.	27	4	1	
Thursday	26. S. W.		4	1	
Friday	27. N. E. & N.		8 ꝺ	0	
Saturday	28. N. E.		10-	1-	infra degel.
	S. S. E.		9-		
Sunday	29. E.		6	0	

T t

March

March	30	Dark weather, pretty windy, no froft; but towards evening a great fall of fnow with a froft, and in the night a ftorm.
Tuefday	31	The wind very high with a froft; but clear and cloudy between whiles.
April	1	For the moft part clear and calm weather, with fome froft.
Thurfday	2	Tolerably calm with fome fnow, but the evening windy, and in the night a violent ftorm.
Friday	3	Stormy, and a fharp froft.
Saturday	4	Clear weather, with fome wind and froft.
Sunday	5	Clear, calm and frofty weather.
Monday	6	Clear and calm weather.
Tuefday	7	Clear, very windy, and a froft.
Wednefday	8	The fame.
Thurfday	9	The fame.
Friday	10	Clear weather, with a little wind and froft.
Saturday	11	Cloudy with fome wind, but no froft.
Sunday	12	Clear, pretty windy, and a froft.
Monday	13	The fame; but in the evening thick and cloudy.
Tuefday	14	Clear, and for the moft part calm weather. During the whole day there was a parhelion, with two mock-funs appearing on each fide, the colours of the rainbow.
Wednefday	15	Clear and calm weather, the evening hazy with fome wind, but no froft.
Thurfday	16	Hazy weather with fome wind; a thaw.
Friday	17	The fame, but lefs wind.
Saturday	18	Thick hazy weather, the wind pretty high, with fome rain.
Sunday	19	The fame.
Monday	20	Clear, calm and mild weather.
Tuefday	21	Hazy weather, with fome wind.
Wednefday	22	For the greater part clear with fome wind.
Thurfday	23	Calm weather with mild fmall rain.
Friday	24	Calm weather, and fine and clear between whiles.
Saturday	25	Clear and calm, but in the night a fharp froft.
Sunday	26	Clear and calm; in the night a froft.

	Wind.	Barom.		Ther.	
March	30. S. W.	26	10	1	fupr. degel.
	N. N. W.				
Tuefday	31. N. N. W.	27	3	2	infra degel.
April	1. N. & E.		6	1	
Thurfday	2. E.		3	1	
	N.	26	11-	3	
Friday	3. N.		11-	3	North light.
Saturday	4. N.	27	4	1	North light.
Sunday	5. E.		6	1	Strong north light.
Monday	6. N.		9	0	
Tuefday	7. N. E.	28	0	0	
Wednefday	8. N. E.	27	7-	1	
Thurfday	9. N. E.		9	1	
Friday	10. N. E.		9	1	
Saturday	11. S. E.		5	1	fupr. degel.
Sunday	12. N. N. E.		6	0	
Monday	13. N. N. E.		11-	2	infra degel.
Tuefday	14. N. E.	28	1	1	
Wednefday	15. E.	27	11	1	fupr. degel.
	S. E.				
Thurfday	16. S. E.		5-	4	
Friday	17. S. S. E.		5	4	
Saturday	18. S. E.		7	5	
Sunday	19. S. E.		10	5	
Monday	20. S. E.		10	5	
Tuefday	21. S. E.		10-	5	
Wednefday	22. S. E.		10 ◡	5	
Thurfday	23. S. E.		10	5	
Friday	24.	28	1	5	
Saturday	25. E.		3	4	
Sunday	26. N. W.		5 ◡	3	

May

1750.		The weather.

April	27	Cloudy, with some wind.
Tuesday	28	By intervals clear, with a little wind in the after-noon, and in the night a high wind and frost.
Wednesday	29	Clear weather, with some wind and frost.
Thursday	30	Clear and calm.
May	1	The same.
Saturday	2	Between whiles gentle showers of rain, and a little wind.
Sunday	3	Clear, calm and mild.
Monday	4	Calm, and between whiles mild rain.
Tuesday	5	Small rain and little wind, but towards the eve-ning clear with high wind.
Wednesday	6	Clear and calm.
Thursday	7	Cloudy with some rain, and the wind pretty high ; but towards evening clear, and a sharp frost.
Friday	8	Clear, the wind high, and some frost.
Saturday.	9	Clear, calm weather with frost; but the after-noon cloudy with wind and rain.
Sunday	10	Cloudy, but for the most part calm.
Monday	11	Between whiles rain and high wind.
Tuesday	12	Cloudy, but calm weather.
Wednesday	13	By intervals gentle showers of rain and a little wind.
Thursday	14	Cloudy and tolerably mild.
Friday	15	Cloudy with a high wind.
Saturday	16	The same, with some rain.
Sunday	17	The same.
Monday	18	Dark weather and pretty windy ; towards the evening clear and calm, and in the night a high wind and rain.
Tuesday	19	Cloudy and windy.
Wednesday	20	The same.
Thursday	21	The same.
Friday	22	Cloudy with some wind ; towards night the wind very high.
Saturday	23	Clear by intervals, and very high wind.
Sunday	24	The same.

	Wind.	Barom.	Ther.	
April	27. S. W.	3	4	
Tuesday	28. S. W.	1 ʊ	4	
Wednesday	29. N.		1	
Thursday	30. N.	2 ʊ	1	
May	1. N.	2	2	
Saturday	2. N. to W.	3	3	
Sunday	3. S. W.	2-	5	
Monday	4. N. W.	3	6	
Tuesday	5. S. W.	4 ʊ	6	
	S. W.	0	6	
Wednesday	6. N. W.			
Thursday	7. N. W.	3	5	
	S. W.	27 10	5	
	N.			
Friday	8. N.	28 0	–	
Saturday	9. N.	2	1	
	S. W.	1	3	
Sunday	10. S.	0 ʊ	5	
Monday	11. W.	27 11	4	
Tuesday	12. W.	28 2	5	
Wednesday	13. S. W.	2-	5	supr. degel.
Thursday	14. S. W.	2	5-	
Friday	15. S. S. E.	3	6	
Saturday	16. S.	3	6	
Sunday	17. S. S. E.	2-	6	
Monday	18. S.	1	7	
		2		
Tuesday	19. S.	0	6	
	till after.	2		
Wednesday	20. S.	3-	6	
Thursday	21. S.	3 ʊ	6	
Friday	22. S. to E.	3	8	
	S. E.			
Saturday	23. S. E.	3	7	
Sunday	24. S. E.	3	7	

U u

May

1750.		The weather.
May	25	Hazy with some rain, but calm.
Tuesday	26	Rain and wind.
Wednesday	27	Clear, calm and warm weather.
Thursday	28	Hazy, but calm weather with small rain.
Friday	29	Clear weather, and pretty windy.
Saturday	30	Clear with some wind.
Sunday	31	The same.
June	1	Driving clouds and a little wind.
Tuesday	2	Clear weather with a little wind.
Wednesday	3	Clear weather with some wind.
Thursday	4	The same.
Friday	5	The same, with very little wind.
Saturday	6	Thick hazy weather with some wind.
Sunday	7	Driving clouds, and between whiles clear, and pretty windy.
Monday	8	Hazy weather, with some rain and wind.
Tuesday	9	Thick hazy weather, with rain and more wind.
Wednesday	10	For the most part clear and pretty windy; but in the night a storm.
Thursday	11	The same; but towards the evening a calm.
Friday	12	The same, with a little wind.
Saturday	13	Clear weather with a little wind.
Sunday	14	Rainy, but calm weather.
Monday	15	Clear weather with some wind.
Tuesday	16	Between whiles clear with some wind.
Wednesday	17	Clear weather and pretty windy.
Thursday	18	The same, with less wind.
Friday	19	Clear, and for the most part calm.
Saturday	20	The same.
Sunday	21	The same.
Monday	22	The same.
Tuesday	23	The same.
Wednesday	24	The same.
Thursday	25	Clear and calm weather.
Friday	26	Cloudy and calm weather.
Saturday	27	Clear and calm weather.
Sunday	28	The same.

Wind.	Barom.	Ther.	
May 25.		3-	8	
Tuefday 26. S.		2	8	
Wednefday 27.		4.	10	
Thurfday 28. N. W.		5	8	
Friday 29. N.		4-	6	
Saturday 30. N. W.		2	6	
Sunday 31. N.	27 11-	6 ᴗ	
June 1. E.to N.&S.	10 ᴗ	6 ᴗ	
Tuefday 2. S. & N.		9-	7	
Wednefday 3. N. W.		9-	8	
Thurfday 4. N. W.		10-	8	
Friday 5. N. W.	28 2	8	
Saturday 6. S.		1	8	
Sunday 7. S. to E.		1-	9	
Monday 8. S.	27 10-	8	
Tuefday 9. S. W.	27 5-	7	fupr. degel.
Wednefday 10. N. E.		8	8 ᴗ	
N. E.		8	5	
Thurfday 11. N. E.		8-	5	
S. E.				
Friday 12. N.		9 ᴗ	6	
Saturday 13. N.		9-	8	
Sunday 14. S. W.		10 ᴗ	9	
Monday 15. S.		11 ᴗ	8	
Tuefday 16. N.		11-	8	
Wednefday 17. N.		11-	8	Holm. fhip.
Thurfday 18. N.	28 0	8-	
Friday 19. N. W.		1 ᴗ	9	
Saturday 20. N W.		2	9	
Sunday 21. N. W.		1•	9	Hafnef. fhip.
Monday 22. N. W.		1	9	
Tuefday 23. W.S.W.&N.	0	10	
Wednefday 24. N.W &W.t S.	27 10-	10	
Thurfday 25. N. E. & S.		11	10	
Friday 26. S. W.	28 0	10	
Saturday 27. N. W.		1	10	
Sunday 28. N. W.		0 ᴗ	11	

May

June	29	Clear weather, and the wind high.
Tuesday	30	The same.
July	1	The same, but pretty calm.
Thursday	2	The same.
Friday	3	The same.
Sunday	19	Hazy weather with some rain and wind.
Monday	20	Pretty clear and calm.
Tuesday	21	The same.
Wednesday	22	Between whiles clear, with a little wind.
Thursday	23	Some rain and a little wind.
Friday	24	Thick hazy weather, but somewhat calm.
Saturday	25	The same.
Sunday	26	Clear weather with a little wind, and in the afternoon some rain.
Monday	27	Clear, with some wind.
Tuesday	28	Cloudy, with a little wind.
Wednesday	29	Between whiles rain and a high wind.
Thursday	30	Dark weather, with a little wind.
Friday	31	High wind with some rain.
August	1	Pretty clear and calm weather.
Sunday	2	Thick hazy weather, and a little windy.
Monday	3	Pretty clear with some wind.
Tuesday	4	The same.
Wednesday	5	Clear weather with a little wind.
Thursday	6	Much the same.
Friday	7	A little rain, but for the most part calm.
Saturday	8	Clear weather and pretty windy.
Sunday	9	The same, with less wind.
Monday	10	The same.
Tuesday	11	Clear and calm weather.
Wednesday	12	The same.
Thursday	13	Clear weather with a very high wind.
Friday	14	Clear and calm weather during almost the whole day.
Saturday	15	The same.
Sunday	16	For the most part clear weather, with a high wind.
Monday	17	By intervals clear, with some wind.

	Wind.	Barom.		Ther.	
June	29. N. W.		0-	10	
Tuesday	30. N. W.		2	10	
July	1. N. W.		6-	11	
Thursday	2. N. W.		5-	11	
Friday	3. N. W.		4-	12	
Sunday	19. E.	27	9	13	
Monday	20. E. & N.		9	13	
Tuesday	21. N W.		9-	13	
Wednesday	22. W.	28	0-	13	
Thursday	23. W. to S.	27	8	12	
Friday	24. W.		5-	12	
Saturday	25. S. W.		5-	12	
Sunday	26. E.		5-.	11-	
	N. E.				
Monday	27. N.		7	9 ̇	
Tuesday	28. N. W.		11.̇	9	
Wednesday	29. S.	28	0	10 ̇	
Thursday	30. S.	28	1 ̇	10	
Friday	31. S. E.	27	9-	10	
August	1. S. & W.		9	10	
Sunday	2. W. & N. W.		9	10	
Monday	3. N.		10 ̇	10	
Tuesday	4. N. W.		11.̇	9	
Wednesday	5. N.		11-	9	
Thursday	6. N.	28	0	9	
Friday	7. S. to E.		1	10	North light.
Saturday	8. N.		2 ̇	10	
Sunday	9. E.	27	11-	10-	
Monday	10. N.		9-	10-	
Tuesday	11. N.		9	10	
Wednesday	12. N. W.		9	11	
Thursday	13. N.		9-	10	
Friday	14.		8-	11	
Saturday	15. E.		8	11	
Sunday	16. N.		8-	10	
Monday	17. S. E.		10-.	11 ̇	

August

1750.   The weather.

Auguſt	18	For the moſt part clear and calm weather.
Wedneſday	19	The ſame, but with ſome wind.
Thurſday	20	Clear and calm.
Friday	21	The ſame.
Saturday	22	The ſame, but foggy.
Sunday	23	Clear and calm weather, towards the evening hazy, with a little rain and wind.
Monday	24	Clear weather with ſome wind.
Thurſday	27	Pretty clear, with a little wind.
Friday	28	Cloudy, with a high wind and a little rain.
Saturday	29	The ſame, but no rain.
Sunday	30	The ſame.
Monday	31	Stormy weather and rain.
September	1	Pretty windy and ſome rain, but in the afternoon clear, with a little wind.
Wedneſday	2	Clear with ſome wind.
Thurſday	3	Cloudy, and a high wind.
Friday	4	The ſame.
Saturday	5	Stormy weather, with the clouds driving.
Sunday	6	Clear and cold weather, and pretty windy.
Monday	7	Wind and rain, but between whiles clear.
Tueſday	8	For the greater part clear with a little wind, and in the mountains ſome ſnow; towards the evening the barometer ſtood.
Wedneſday	9	A continual rain, and pretty high wind.
Thurſday	10	Clouds, with a pretty high wind; by intervals clear, and in the night a froſt.
Friday	11	Clear and calm, towards evening a little wind.
Saturday	12	Rain and wind; but between whiles clear.
Sunday	13	Rain and a pretty deal of wind.
Monday	14	The ſame; at noon the rain ceaſed, and the weather was calm and mild.
Tueſday	15	The wind very high with ſome rain; afternoon very rainy and windy.
Wedneſday	16	Cloudy and pretty windy.
Thurſday	17	Cloudy, but for the moſt part calm; in the afternoon a little ſmall rain, and quite calm; but rain during almoſt the whole night.

	Wind.	Barom.	Ther.	
Auguft	18. S. E. & N.E.	11-	11-	
Wednefday	19. N. E.	10-	11	
Thurfday	20.	9-	11	North light.
Friday	21. N.	9-	11	
Saturday	22. N. W.	9-	11	
Sunday	23. S. E.	27 9-	11-	
	S. E.			
Monday	24. E.	9-	11-	
Thurfday	27. S. W.	11-	11	
Friday	28. S. S. E.	28 0 ʋ	10-	
Saturday	29. E.	27 7-	10	
Sunday	30. E. to S.	6 ʋ	10	
Monday	31. S. E. S. to W.	3-	10	
September	1. S. E.	4	10	
	N. E. & N.	6	10 ʋ	
Wednefday	2. N. & W.	9	9	North light.
Thurfday	3. E.	2 ʋ	9-	
Friday	4. N. E. & N.	2-	8 ʋ	
Saturday	5. N. E.	7	6	
Sunday	6. N.	9-	6	Strong north light.
Monday	7. S.	10-	8	
Tuefday	8. N. W.	10-	8	
		28 0		
Wednefday	9. S. to W.	27 8	9	
Thurfday	10. W. S. W.	7-	6-	
Friday	11. S. to E.	9-	6-	Strong north light.
Saturday	12. S. to W.	9	8	
Sunday	13. S E. & S.	8-	8	
Monday	14. S.	7-	9	
	W.	11		
Tuefday	15. S. E.	11-	8-	
		9-		
Wednefday	16. S. to E.	28 0	10	
Thurfday	17. S. to E.	1	10	

September

1750.   The weather.

September	18	Cloudy and the wind pretty high; in the afternoon a little rain.
Saturday	19	Cloudy and pretty windy.
Sunday	20	Showery with fome wind; but in the night a calm and continual rain.
Monday	21	Rain and calm weather; but the evening windy, and a violent ftorm in the night.
Tuefday	22	Stormy, fhowery, and between whiles fun-fhine.
Wednefday	23	Showery, windy, and by intervals fun-fhine, and the wind pretty ftill.
Thurfday	24	Somewhat windy and fhowery, but towards the evening clear and windy.
Friday	25	Rainy weather, but fomewhat calm.
Saturday	26	Unfettled weather, rain, fun-fhine, and very windy.
Sunday	27	Foggy, but calm, in the evening and night a violent ftorm and rain.
Monday	28	Cloudy and windy; during the afternoon rain, and fnow in the mountains.
Tuefday	29	Clear and windy, with fhowers of rain and hail.
Wednefday	30	Windy and fhowery.
October	1	Rainy and windy.
Friday	2	Thick hazy weather and windy; in the evening a high wind and rain.
Saturday	3	At eight o'clock, A. M. calm and clear, about noon heavy rain and fome wind; in the afternoon fome fhowers of rain, and between whiles fun-fhine.
Sunday	4	By intervals clear, fhowery and windy; but during the evening and night, continual rain and calm.
Monday	5	Pretty windy and fhowery; in the afternoon and evening, an almoft conftant rain and wind.
Tuefday	6	A continual fmall rain, but the weather fomewhat calm, and the air dark and foggy.
Wednefday	7	Between whiles clear and fome wind.
Thurfday	8	A continual rain and wind.
Friday	9	Clear and windy, in the night froft and fnow.
Saturday	10	A very high wind, accompanied with hail.
Sunday	11	Cloudy and calm, with a little froft.
Monday	12	The fame, but clearer and no froft.

1750.

	Wind.	Barom.	Ther. open air.	
September	18. S S. E.	1	10c	
		0-		
Saturday	19. E. S. E.	27 11-	10 ᴜ	
Sunday	20. S. W. & S.	9	10 ᴜ	
Monday	21. S. E.	5	9	
	N. E.	1		
Tuefday	22. S. E.	3-	8 ᴜ	
Wednefday	23. E. S. E.	6-	8	Str. north light.
Thurfday	24. E. S. E.	5-	7	
	N.	4-	7 ᴜ	
Friday	25. N. E. & W.	2	7	
Saturday	26. S. & S. to E.	7	7 ᴜ	
Sunday	27. S. to E.	9	7	
	N. W.	5	6	
Monday	28. W.	3	6	
	N. W.	4	5-	
Tuefday	29. S. W.	6	5	
Wednefday	30. S.	3	5	
October	1. N. E. & N.	3	5	
Friday	2. E.	5	5	
	E. to N.	26 11		
Saturday	3. S.	27 10 ᴜ		
		10-	6 ᴜ	
		28 0		
Sunday	4. S. W.	3-	7 ᴜ	
		6		
Monday	5. S. W.	7	7	
	W. S. W.	7-	7-	
Tuefday	6. S. W.	8	7-	
Wednefday	7. S. W.	6	7 ᴜ	
Thurfday	8. S.	3	7 ᴜ	
Friday	9. W.toS.&N.W.	0	7 ᴜ	North light.
Saturday	10. W.	27 11	4	1 fupr. degel.
Sunday	11. N. & N. E.	28 2	3	0 North light.
Monday	12. S. W.	5		3

Y y   October

1750.   The weather.

October	13	Rainy and windy, and the air thick and hazy.
Wednefday	14	The air thick and hazy, with fome fhowers, but towards the evening clear.
Thurfday	15	Cloudy with fome wind and fhowers; in the night it fnowed in the mountains.
Friday	16	Clear and calm; but in the night a ftorm.
Saturday	17	Stormy weather with heavy fhowers, and about ten o'clock, P. M. a violent ftorm.
Sunday	18	Stormy weather, between whiles clear, but in the night a moft violent ftorm.
Monday	19	Stormy and fhowery; at midnight the ftorm abated.
Tuefday	20	Windy and fhowery; at noon it began to be calm.
Wednefday	21	By intervals clear, and for the moft part calm.
Thurfday	22	The fame.

The glade of the north-light paffed from E. N. E. to W. N. W. through the zenith extremely lucid, and many fmall radii, though not fo bright, fhot the fame way, all from the north, but none from the fouth. About nine o'clock the fky was covered with clouds, and after hardly any north light appeared in the clouds.

Friday	23	Light clouds, and calm weather.
Saturday	24	Between whiles clear, but for the moft part calm.
Sunday	25	For the moft part clear and calm, in the night a froft.
Monday	26	Clear and calm. In the evening of this day two luminous arches were feen to the fouth, about 16 degrees above the horizon, being the point from whence the direction of their rays was towards the zenith between S. E. and S. W. With all the celerity of an inftantaneous motion, rays gufhed forth on both fides to the Eaft and Weft, and ftood collected about the zenith. From thence they darted towards the other hemifphere, and for fome time made a moft beautiful appearance, like a glory or

circle

	Wind.	Barom.	Ther. open air.	
October	13. S.		3	7	
Wednesday	14. S. & W.	27	11	6	
Thursday	15. S. W. & W.		9	4-	
Friday	16. S. to E.	28	0-	3-	
	S. E.	27	10		
Saturday	17. S. E.		9	6	
			8 ᴏ		
Sunday	18. S. E.		9-	5	
Monday	19. S. E.		10 ᴏ	5	
Tuesday	20. S. to E.		11	6	
	S.				Str. north light.
Wednesday	21. S.	28	1	6	
Thursday	22. S.		2-	5	Str. north light.
			3	4	
Friday	23. S. E.		4 ᴏ	5	North light.
Saturday	24. S.		3	5-	North light.
Sunday	25. S. E.		5-	6	North light.
Monday	26. S. E.		5	1	Str. north light.

October

circle of effulgent beams. Afterwards this north light extended its corrufcations farther to the North, and therein formed an arch of about 24 degrees altitude. In the beginning of the evening till paft 7 o'clock, no ftreams of the light appeared in the North, but it after continued the remainder of the evening as ufual, with very bright arches interfecting the zenith from Eaft to Weft. The ftar-light was very corrufcant, and the evening fine and clear.

October	27	Clear and calm weather, with a little froft. The north-light appeared prefently after the fun-fet as ufual, with a ftrong bright bow or arch, from Eaft to Weft, which ftreamed like a river from Weft to Eaft. It is thus it commonly appears, except when rays dart from the North or South. Towards 7 o'clock, it grew fo dark, that the ftars could hardly be perceived.
Wednefday	28	The forenoon was clear; about noon light clouds appeared, with calm weather and a little froft. The night before there was a pretty hard froft.
Thurfday	29	Small rain but calm.
Friday	30	Some rain and a little wind; in the evening and night a froft.
Saturday	31	Clear calm weather with a froft.
November	1	The fame, with a little wind.
Monday	2	The fame.
Tuefday	3	Cloudy but calm, without any froft.
Wednefday	4	Clear with fome wind and froft.
Thurfday	5	Clear with a little wind and froft. A fog in the evening.
Friday	6	Clear, windy and frofty.
Saturday	7	Clear and calm, with a little froft.
Sunday	8	Clear, with a little wind and froft.
Monday	9	Clear and calm, with a little froft; towards evening hazy, and a little fnow.
Tuefday	10	Clear weather, with a little wind and froft.

	Wind.	Barom.	Ther. open air.

		Wind.		Barom.		Ther.	
October	27.	S. E.					
Wednesday	28.	S. E.		4		2	
Thursday	29.	S.E. & N.W.		4		2-	North light.
Friday	30.	N. W. & N.		3-		2 ᴗ	North light.
Saturday	31.	E.		4-		o	North light.
November	1	N.		5		2-	infra degel.
Monday	2.	E.		5		2	North light.
Tuesday	3.	N.		4		3	supr. degel.
Wednesday	4.	E.		4		o	St. flying nor. light.
Thursday	5.	E. & N. E.	28	3		2-	Strong north light. infra degel.
Friday	6.	N. E.		2-		2-	North light.
Saturday	7.	S. E.		2 ᴗ		2 ᴗ	North light.
Sunday	8.	N.t.W.&N.		1		2	North light.
Monday	9.	S. E.	27	11		1-	North light.
Tuesday	10.	E.		10		o	

Z z   November

1750.		The weather.

November	11	Hazy weather and pretty windy, but no froft; the evening calm, with fome rain and fnow.
Thurfday	12	Hazy weather with fome wind; the afternoon very windy and rainy, at 9 o'clock, P. M. clear and calm.
Friday	13	Clear and calm, in the afternoon rain, and in the night a ftorm with a little froft.
Saturday	14	Stormy yet clear, with fome froft; the ftorm continued all the evening.
Sunday	15	Stormy, but for the moft part clear, with fome froft; the afternoon and evening calm, though hazy, and without froft.
Monday	16	Clear and calm weather; the evening the fame.
Tuefday	17	Foggy but calm.
Wednefday	18	Hazy, mild and calm weather.
Thurfday	19	Foggy, with a little wind.
Friday	20	The fame, with fome fhowers of rain.
Saturday	21	The fame, but for the moft part calm.
Sunday	22	The fame, but with a continual fmall rain.
Monday	23	The fame.
Tuefday	24	The fame.
Wednefday	25	The fame, with a little wind, and in the night fome froft.
Thurfday	26	By intervals clear, fome wind and froft.
Friday	27	For the moft part clear, with a little wind and froft; in the night fnow.
Saturday	28	Hazy, with fome wind and froft; towards evening a high wind and rain, but no froft.
Sunday	29	Clear weather, with fome wind and a froft.
Monday	30	Clear and calm with fome froft.
December	1	Hazy, a little wind, but no froft.
Wednefday	2	Rainy, and pretty windy.
Thurfday	3	Hazy, fhowery, and a high wind.
Friday	4	Hazy, with fome wind but no rain; in the afternoon clear and calm weather, and in the night a little froft.
Saturday	5	Cloudy, fome wind, no froft, and in the evening a ftorm. 1750.

	Wind.	Barom.	Ther. open air.	
November	11. S.	11 ᴗ	1	fupr. degel.
Thurſday	12. E.	9		
	S. E. & S.	6-	3	
	S.	4-		
Friday	13. E.	4-		
	S. E.		2	
Saturday	14. N. E.			
	N. E.	5	1	infra degel.
		8-		
Sunday	15. N E.	11	1	North light.
	E.	28 2	3	infra degel.
Monday	16. S. S. E.	5-		
		6	1 ᴗ	North light.
Tueſday	17. N.	8	2 ᴗ	fupr. degel.
Wedneſday	18.	9	4	North light.
Thurſday	19. W.	7-	4-	North light.
Friday	20. S. W.	4-	5 ᴗ	
Saturday	21. W.	4-	4-	North light.
Sunday	22. S. W.	3	4	North light.
Monday	23. S. W.	4	4	North light.
Tueſday	24. S. W.	4	4	North light.
Wedneſday	25. W.	1	4	North light.
Thurſday	26. E.	4 ᴗ	2	infra degel.
Friday	27. S. E.	5 ᴗ	2-	North light.
				North light.
Saturday	28. S. S. E.			
	S.	28 0 ᴗ	2-	fupr. degel.
Sunday	29. N.	2	0-	infra degel.
Monday	30. E. to S.	5-	3-	Strong north light.
December	1. S. E.	3-	3	fupr. degel.
Wedneſday	2. S.	27 9-	6	
Thurſday	3. S. to W.	8 ᴗ	5-	
Friday	4. W.	11		
	W. to N.	28 2 ᴗ	2 ᴗ	North light.
Saturday	5. S. E.			
		27 9-	4-	December

Before the ſtorm began, the moon had cloſe round it a halo, or ring of the colours of a rainbow, about a hand's breadth in appearance, and oval according to the ſhape of the moon, which then was almoſt in the firſt quarter. About this halo was another of the ſame breadth, exceeding luminous and clear. Preſently after the appearance of this meteor, it grew very cloudy, and the ſtorm began, and did not ceaſe till towards morning.

December 6 — Cloudy, ſhowery, windy, a large halo round the moon, and a great ſtorm in the night about 24 hours after the former was allayed.

Monday 7 — A ſtorm with hail and rain; about noon the ſtorm ceaſing, it continued a little windy, with a few ſtrong guſts by intervals.

Tueſday 8 — In the forenoon rain and wind; but the afternoon clear and calm, and a froſt in the night.

Wedneſday 9 — Clear and calm with a little froſt; in the afternoon and evening pretty high wind.

Thurſday 10 — Clear and calm, with a little froſt.

Friday 11 — Clear with ſome wind and a froſt; the afternoon and evening pretty windy.

Saturday 12 — Cloudy, and a high wind about ſeven o'clock, A. M.

Sunday 13 — Calm clear weather, and a froſt; in the evening a great halo round the moon.

Monday 14 — Clear and calm with a froſt.
Tueſday 15 — The ſame.
Wedneſday 16 — The ſame.

It is remarkable, that though calm and clear weather had continued now upwards of five days, except a little wind the 11th and 12th, yet the barometer was very low, and at ſea there was ſuch ruffling hard north weather, that they could not row five or ſix miles out at ſea to fiſh, before they met with ſwelling ſurges, the noiſe of which might be heard from the ſhore.

1750.

Wind.		Barom.		Ther. open air.
December	6. S.	27 9	1-	fupr. degel.
Monday	7. E.	0-	4-	North light.
Tuefday	8. S. to E.	5-	2 0	North light.
Wednefday	9. E.	5-		infra degel.
	N. E.	3-	0-	North light.
Thurfday	10. E.	2-	2 0	North light.
Friday	11. N. E.	3 0		
	N.		2-	
Saturday	12. N.	3	2	North light.
			4	
Sunday	13. S. to E.	3-	3-	North light.
Monday	14. S. E.	27 6	4 0	infra degel.
Tuefday	15. S. E.	5 0	4	North light.
Wednefday	16. S. to E.	7-	5	Strong north light.
				North light.

A a a   December

1750.		The weather.

December	17	Clouds driving, pretty windy, and a froft.
Friday	18	Cloudy, windy and frofty; towards evening fnow.
Saturday	19	The forenoon cloudy, but the afternoon clear, calm and frofty.
Sunday	20	Snow, with wind and froft; towards the evening rain and wind, but no froft.
Monday	21	Clouds but calm and fhowery; froft in the night.
Tuefday	22	Hazy, towards the evening rain, but for the moft part calm; in the night a froft.
Wednefday	23	Cloudy, between whiles clear, but for the moft part calm, with a little froft.
Thurfday	24	Very high wind and rain.
Friday	25	Cloudy, with a little wind, and in the evening fome froft.
Saturday	26	In the forenoon wind, fnow and froft; but in the afternoon calm, towards the evening rain, and in the night a high wind and froft.
Sunday	27	Stormy, but by intervals clear and frofty; The evening quite calm with a froft.
Monday	28	Hazy, windy and rainy.
Tuefday	29	Cloudy, but for the moft part calm and mild weather.
Wednefday	30	Hazy, windy and rainy.
Thurfday	31	The fame, but lefs wind.
1751.		
January	1	Foggy, but for the moft part calm. The evening was pretty clear, and had a ftrong north light all over the fky, but chiefly in the fouth and about the zenith. No rays proceeding from the north, except about the zenith. At half an hour paft 10, P. M. it grew hazy, as it ufually does after the north light.

	Wind.	Barom.	Ther. open air.	
December	17. N.	10 ᴜ	5-	North light.
Friday	18. E.	9-		
			0-	
Saturday	19. E.	9-	4-	North light.
Sunday	20. N.	4	4	
	E.	0	2-	fupra degel.
Monday	21. E. to S.	26 10-	2	
	N. E.			
Tuefday	22. N. E.	27 1-	2	
Wednefday	23. S.	27 8	1 ᴜ	
Thurfday	24. S.	7	2	
Friday	25. N. W.	9-		North light.
	N.		0-	
Saturday	26. N.	8		
	E.	5-	1	
	N.			
Sunday	27. N.	10-	4-	infra degel. Strong north light. At 11 o'clock, P.M. it grew hazy, but no froft.
		28 4 ᴜ		
Monday	28. S.	2	2-	fupr. degel.
Tuefday	29. S.	1	3	
Wednefday	30. S	0	3	
Thurfday	31. S. & S. E.	2 ᴜ	4	
1751.				
January	1. S.	28 1	1	fupr. degel.

		Froſt in the night.
January	2	No froſt, but cloudy, with a little wind.
		In the evening it was clear, and a ſtrong north light appeared about half an hour paſt five, as alſo an arch or bow in the North, which roſe gradually to the zenith, and afterwards in a direction to the South, where between whiles three broad arches from Eaſt to Weſt were very corruſcant, but ſtood clear and luminous without ſcintillations.
Sunday	3	Hazy and calm with rain; but in the night a little froſt.
Monday	4	Hazy, and for the moſt part calm with ſome froſt; in the evening a pretty ſtrong north light to the ſouth.
Tueſday	5	The forenoon clear, very windy and a froſt; in the afternoon the wind much higher, and the froſt ſharper; in the evening a north light.
Wedneſday	6	Clear weather and a high wind, at ſix o'clock, P. M. calm, and afterwards a north light.
Thurſday	7	Forenoon clear and calm, with a ſharp froſt; the afternoon hazy with leſs froſt.
Friday	8	For the moſt part clear, with a little wind and froſt; in the evening a very high wind, froſt, and north light.
Saturday	9	Clear, ſtormy and a froſt; in the afternoon hazy.
Sunday	10	Somewhat hazy, with a very high wind and froſt; in the evening leſs wind, but clearer and a froſt.
Monday	11	Between whiles clear, with a high wind and froſt.
Tueſday	12	Hazy, pretty windy, and a froſt.
Wedneſday	13	Hazy, pretty windy, and no froſt; in the evening rain and leſs wind.
Thurſday	14	Rain and hail with ſome wind; but in the evening pretty clear, a froſt and north lights, and in the night ſnow.
Friday	15	Hazy weather, pretty windy, and no froſt; in the afternoon and evening ſtormy and ſhowery; and in the night exceeding ſtormy.

	Wind.	Barom.	Ther. open air.	
January	2. S.	27 11	1	
Sunday	3. S. S. W.	8-	3	
Monday	4. S. W.	8-	2	infra degel. North light.
Tuesday	5. N.	8- 11-	9	North light.
Wednesday	6. N.	28 1 2-	9 10	North light.
Thursday	7. S. E.	2 1 ʊ	10 5 ʊ	
Friday	8. E. S. E. N.	1 2	4 ʊ 6	North light.
Saturday	9. N.	27 11	4 ʊ	
Sunday	10. N. N. E.	9 8-	2- 5	
Monday	11. N.	27 5	6	infra degel.
Tuesday	12. E.	3 ʊ	1	
Wednesday	13. S. E. S.	26 11 ʊ	4	supra degel.
Thursday	14. W. N. W.	27 1- 3 ʊ	2 o-	infra degel. North light.
Friday	15. S. E.	3- -o- 26 9-	4-	supr. degel.

B b b   January

January	16	Towards noon the storm abated, towards evening quite calm, hazy, and a little snow.
Sunday	17	Between whiles clear, calm, and a little frost.
Monday	18	Hazy, with a little snow, frost and wind; in the evening pretty calm weather and a north light.
Tuesday	19	By intervals clear and hazy, with a high wind, hail, snow, and a little frost.
Wednesday	20	The forenoon hazy and calm, between whiles snow; in the evening a storm and rain, which lasted three or four hours; afterwards a moderate wind.
Thursday	21	By intervals calm, showery and windy; the evening pretty clear, with a little frost and a north light.
Friday	22	Between whiles clear with some snow, no great wind, and a little frost; the evening calm, with a strong north light.
Saturday	23	Hazy, with some wind and frost; in the afternoon high winds and snow; in the evening a storm, afterwards clear, with a sharp frost, and north light.
Sunday	24	Clear, with a high wind and frost; the wind abated in the evening about eight o'clock, at which time there was a strong north light in the north.
Monday	25	Clear and calm weather; with a sharp frost; at noon and in the afternoon, till 4 o'clock; the evening hazy and calm about nine o'clock.
Tuesday	26	Hazy, calm and frosty; in the afternoon snow and a high wind, in the night a storm, and a sharp frost.
Wednesday	27	Clear weather, with a high wind and frost; in the afternoon the wind abated; in the evening clear, calm and a frost, and in the night a high wind.

	Wind.	Barom.	Ther. open air.	
January	16. S. E. A. M.	9-		
		27 1-	1 0	
Sunday	17. S. E. & E.	1	0	
Monday	18. S. to E.	4-	o-	infra degel. North light.
Tuesday	19. S. to W. & E.	5-	o-	
Wednesday	20. S.	7	0	
	S. clock 11	2-	3	supr. degel.
Thursday	21. S.	2	o-	infra degel. North light.
Friday	22. S. W. & S.	o-	1-	
Saturday	23. E. N E.	1-		North light.
	N.	6	7	North light.
Sunday	24. N.	11-	10	North light.
Monday	25. S. E.	28 0	11 13 9-	
Tuesday	26. E. N. E.	27 9	5 clock	infra degel.
Wednesday	27. N.	9 28 0	12 7- 9-	

January	28	Clear with high wind and froft; in the evening a ftorm, and ftrong north light, and in the night a very great ftorm.
Friday	29	Stormy, fomewhat hazy, and a froft.
Saturday	30	Hazy, ftormy, and a little froft; in the night the wind laid itfelf.
Sunday	31	Clear and calm weather with a little froft; in the evening a ftrong north light in the fouth.
February	1	Hazy, but for the moft part calm and mild weather.
Tuefday	2	Hazy, with fmall rain and fome wind.
Wednefday	3	Hazy and calm, with continual rain; in the night a high wind and froft.
Thurfday	4	Clear weather, pretty windy, and a froft; the afternoon for the moft part calm with a froft, but the evening fomewhat hazy and calm.
Friday	5	Hazy and calm, with a little froft; in the evening a large but faint halo round the moon, and in the night a ftorm and fharp froft.
Saturday	6	Clear but ftormy, with a fharp froft.
Sunday	7	The fame; in the evening fnow and lefs wind, but in the night a ftorm.
Monday	8	Clear weather, but ftormy and frofty; in the evening the ftorm abated.
Tuefday	9	Hazy, and for the moft part calm, with fome fnow and rain; towards evening a high wind, and between whiles fnow and rain.
Wednefday	10	By intervals clear, calm and hazy, with wind and froft; in the evening lefs wind, but cloudy.
Thurfday	11	Clear and calm weather with a froft; in the evening a north light in the fouth.
Friday	12	Hazy and calm with a froft; the evening clear, with a faint north light.
Saturday	13	For the moft part calm and clear with fome froft; towards evening hazy, but a north light in the fouth.
Sunday	14	Hazy weather, with fome wind and a little froft.
Monday	15	Hazy with fnow and wind; the evening calm, without fnow, but frofty.

	Wind.	Barom.	Ther. open air.	
January	28. N E.	27 11-		
		10-	8-	North light.
Friday	29. N. E.	7	3	
Saturday	30. N. E.	7	0	
Sunday	31. E.	28 2		
			1	North light.
February	1. S. to E.	2-	3 ◡	fupr. degel.
Tuefday	2. S. to E.	27 11-	4	
Wednefday	3. S. to E.	11-	4	
	N. N. E.			
Thurfday	4. N. N. E.	28 3 ◡	1 ◡	infra degel.
	E.	6 ◡	1-	
Friday	5. E.	3-	1-	
	N.			
Saturday	6. N.	4	9	
Sunday	7. N.	4-	9	
Monday	8. N.	4-	7-	
Tuefday	9. E. & S.	5-		
	N.	4	9-	
Wednefday	10. N. & N. E.	1 ◡	6	
	E.	3-	1-	
Thurfday	11. E.	28 5 ◡	4	infra degel.
				North light.
Friday	12. S. E.	4 ◡	2-	
			4-	North light.
Saturday	13. N. E. & E.	2-		
			2	North light.
Sunday	14. E. N E.	1-	0	
Monday	15. E. N. E.			
		27 10-	0	

C c c

1751.		The weather.

February	16	Clear and calm with a froft; in the evening a north light, with ftrong vibrating rays from the north eaft.
Wednefday	17	Hazy, with fome wind and froft.
Thurfday	18	Hazy, and pretty calm, with fome fnow; the evening clear, with a ftrong north light, and arches firft appearing in the fouth, and afterwards in the north.
Friday	19	Foggy, calm, and by intervals clear; the evening calm and rainy.
Saturday	20	Hazy, with fome wind and fhowers; in the afternoon a high wind and rain; the evening calm and clear, with a north light.
Sunday	21	Hazy, with a high wind; the afternoon rainy; but in the evening clear, and a north light.
Monday	22	Rain, and fleet, and a high wind; in the night a little froft.
Tuefday	23	Hazy and calm; the afternoon and evening clear, fhowery, and windy, with a north light to the fouth.
Wednefday	24	Hazy and calm, but in the night a froft.
Thurfday	25	Hazy and quite calm, with a little froft; the evening foggy.
Friday	26	Hazy and calm without a froft; towards evening windy.
Saturday	27	Hazy and fomewhat calm, with a little fnow; the night windy and frofty.
Sunday	28	Cloudy, high wind, but little froft; the evening calm and clear, with a north light in the fouth.
March	1	Clear and calm with froft; in the evening north light in the fouth.
Tuefday	2	Hazy with fome wind and a little froft; in the evening a north light N. E. and N. W. towards the zenith.
Wednefday	3	Clear, calm and frofty; in the evening a ftrong north light, firft in the fouth, afterwards in the north, and then all over the fky.

	Wind.	Barom.	Ther. open air.	
February	16. S. E.	9-	4	
			6-	North light.
Wednesday	17. N. E. & E.	10-	2 ʊ	
Thursday	18. N. E.	10-	0	
		8-	1-	North light.
Friday	19. N. E.	8-	2	
	E.	6	1-	supr. degel.
Saturday	20. E. S. E.	6-		
	E.	5	3 ʊ	North light.
Sunday	21. E.	26 9		
	S. to E.	11 ʊ	4 ʊ	North light.
Monday	22. S & S. W.	27 6-	4	
Tuesday	23. S. & S. W.	7-		
		8-	2	North light.
Wednesday	24. W.	10	2	
Thursday	25.	10-	1 ʊ	supra degel.
Friday	26. S. E.	28 0		
		27 10	2	
Saturday	27. S. & W.	27 7 ʊ	1 ʊ	
	N.			
Sunday	28. N.	4		
		7	2	infra degel.
				North light.
March	1 E.	9	5	North light.
Tuesday	2. E.	7	0	
				North light.
Wednesday	3. S. E. & N.	11 ʊ	5	North light.
			6-	

1751.   The weather.

March	4	Clear weather, pretty windy, and a froft; towards the evening the wind ceafed, and afterwards a ftrong north light appeared chiefly in the fouth.
Friday	5	Hazy weather, very high wind, and a little froft.
Saturday	6	The fame, with fome fhowers.
Sunday	7	Hazy, windy and fhowery; the evening calm, but rainy.
Monday	8	Hazy and windy; in the night a froft.
Tuefday	9	Hazy and calm, but no froft.
Wednefday	10	The fame; in the afternoon rain, and in the night a froft.
Thurfday	11	Hazy, with a little wind.
Friday	12	Hazy and pretty windy.
Saturday	13	The fame; but with fhowers of rain and fnow.
Sunday	14	Hazy and a little windy; towards evening clear and calm, with a little froft.
Monday	15	Hazy and calm; the afternoon and evening windy.
Tuefday	16	Hazy, fhowery and windy.
Wednefday	17	The forenoon clear and calm, but the afternoon and evening hazy and a little wind.
Thurfday	18	Hazy and windy; the evening clear, with lefs wind and a froft.
Friday	19	Hazy, with a little wind; the evening hazy and a little froft.
Saturday	20	Clear weather, with a little wind and froft; in the evening a ftrong north light to the fouth.
Sunday	21	Clear weather with fome wind; the evening calm, and a ftrong north light.
Monday	22	Cloudy, high wind, and a little froft; the evening calm and clear.
Tuefday	23	Hazy, calm and fhowery.
Wednefday	24	Hazy and windy, with fnow and rain.
Thurfday	25	Hazy, with fome wind; the evening hazy and calm, in the night fome fnow fell.
Friday	26	By intervals hazy and clear, but for the moft part calm; the evening clear, with a north light and little froft.

1751.

	Wind.	Barom.	Ther. open air.	
March	4. N.	28 1		
	S. E.			
			8	North light.
Friday	5. E.	27 7	1 o	
Saturday	6. E. & S. E.	0-	4 o	fupr. degel.
Sunday	7. E. to S.	26 -8		
		9	4 o	
Monday	8. E.	9-	3-	
Tuefday	9. E.	27 0-	3-	
Wednefday	10. E.	3-	3-	
Thurfday	11. E.	5 o	2-	
Friday	12. E.	0	2	
Saturday	13. N. E. & E.	26 8-	2	
Sunday	14. N. to E.	10		
	S. E.	11-	1	
Monday	15. E.	27 0		
	N.		2-	
Tuefday	16. E.	5-	3	
Wednefday	17. E.	8-	2-	
Thurfday	18. S. E.			
	E.	9-	1	
Friday	19. N. E. & E.	27 9 o	1	fupr. degel.
Saturday	20. E. to N.	7-	1	infra degel.
			2	North light.
Sunday	21. E. & N.	5-	o	
		3	2	North light.
Monday	22. N.	2-		
		3-	1	
Tuefday	23. E. & S.	5-	2-	fupra degel.
Wednefday	24. E. & E. by S.	3	2	North light.
Thurfday	25. E.	0-		
	S.	2-	3	
Friday	26.			

March	27	Hazy and calm.
Sunday	. 28	Between whiles clear and pretty windy ; in the night a froft and north light.
Monday	29	Hazy with fome wind ; in the night a froft and a little north light.
Tuefday	30	Clear and calm.
Wednefday	31	Clear, windy and frofty ; in the evening a little froft and north light all over the fky.
April	1	Clouds driving, with a little wind, no froft.
Friday	2	Hazy weather, pretty windy and fhowery ; the evening clear and calm, and a north light.
Saturday	3	Hazy, fome wind and rain ; the evening clear and calm with a north light.
Sunday	4	Between whiles clear, and for the moft part calm.
Monday	5	Hazy, fhowery and calm.
Tuefday	6	Between whiles hazy with fnow, but for the moft part calm.
Wednefday	7	Hazy with fome fnow, but calm ; in the night a violent ftorm.
Thurfday	8	Hazy, ftormy, and a froft ; in the evening and night the ftorm greater, and the froft continued.
Friday	9	Hazy, and a violent ftorm with fome froft.
Saturday	10	Between whiles clear, with a high wind and froft ; the evening a little windy.
Sunday	11	Hazy, calm and no froft.
Monday	12	Clear, towards evening windy.
Tuefday	13	Clear, calm and a little froft ; in the evening a ftrong north light, and in the day a great halo round the fun ; the preceding day in the forenoon there was a mock fun, which in the afternoon appeared behind the real.
Wednefday	14	Between whiles clear and calm weather, in the evening a north light.
Thurfday	15	Between whiles clear, with fome wind.
Friday	16	Hazy, and pretty windy.
Saturday	17	Hazy, windy and fhowery ; the wind was very high all the evening and night.

	Wind.	Barom.	Ther. open air.	
March	27. N. E. & E.	5-	0	North light.
Sunday	28. N. E. & E.	5-	1	
Monday	29. N.N.E.&E.	6	2	North light.
Tuefday	30. N. & N. E.	11 ◡	1	
Wednefday	31. N. & S. E.	28 3	0-	North light.
	N.	3-	0	
			2	infra degel.
April	1 S. E.	1-	2	fupr. degel.
Friday	2. S. E. & S.	27 11	2-	North light.
Saturday	3. S.	8 ◡	2-	North light.
Sunday	4. S. E.	6-	2	
Monday	5. S. W. & W.	6	2	
Tuefday	6. S.	4 ◡	2 ◡	
Wednefday	7. N.	1-	2 ◡	
	N.			
Thurfday	8. N.	6	0	
Friday	9. N.	28 0 ◡	3-	infra degel.
Saturday	10. N.	28 2-	3-	
Sunday	11. S. & S. W.	27 9	3-	fupra degel.
Monday	12. S. W. & N. W.	10-	2 ◡	
Tuefday	13. N.	28 2-	1 ◡	infra degel. North light.
Wednefday	14.	2 ◡	2-	fupr. degel. North light.
Thurfday	15. S. to E.	3	4-	
Friday	16. S. S. E.	3-	5	
Saturday	17. S. S. E.	3-	6	

April

April	18	The fame; in the evening hazy and mild weather with fmall rain.
Monday	19	Hazy and rainy, but for the moft part calm.
Tuefday	20	For the moft part hazy and calm.
Wednefday	21	Between whiles clear and calm.
Thurfday	22	The fame.
Friday	23	Pretty clear, with very little wind; the evening mild and clear.
Saturday	24	Hazy and calm with fome fhowers.
Sunday	25	Hazy with fome wind.
Monday	26	Between whiles clear but little wind; evening clear, with a ftrong north light about the zenith.
Tuefday	27	Hazy and calm.
Wednefday	28	Clear and calm; the evening calm and hazy.
Thurfday	29	Clear and a little wind.
Friday	30	The fame.
May	1	Delightful fummer weather; clear with a little wind; the evening bright and ferene.
Sunday	2	The fame; but the evening a little hazy.
Monday	3	Clear and calm; in the evening a few clouds and a north light.
Tuefday	4	Clear, calm and mild weather, with little froft in the night.
Wednefday	5	Hazy and warm weather with fome wind; but a flight froft in the night.
Thurfday	6	The fame; but the evening clear, and a little froft in the night.
Friday	7	Clear and mild; in the evening a little wind.
Saturday	8	Hazy and calm, with fome fhowers.
Sunday	9	Clear, with a high wind that ceafed towards night, during which there was a pretty fharp froft.
Monday	10	For the moft part clear, with a cold wind; in the evening a high chilling wind, and in the night a froft and ftorm.

	Wind.	Barom.	Ther. open air.	
April	18. S. S. E.	2-		
		3-	6	
Monday	19. N.	3-	3	
Tuesday	20. E.	3	6	
Wednesday	21. E.	2 ᴜ	5	
Thursday	22. E.	27 10	3-	
Friday	23. E. & N. E.	8-		
	N. E.	28 0 ᴜ	3-	
Saturday	24. S. E.	3	4	
Sunday	25. S. E.	2 ᴜ	5	
Monday	26. N. W.	2	3 ᴜ	North light.
Tuesday	27. W. & N.W.	5 ᴜ	4-	
Wednesday	28. N. by W. & E.	4		
			3-	
Thursday	29. N. W.	3-	4-	Evening.
Friday	30. N. W.	3	5	Evening.
May	1 N.	3	9-	
			4	Evening.
Sunday	2. W.	5 ᴜ	8	
	S.		4-	Evening.
Monday	3. N. W.			
	S.	28 5-	5 ᴜ	
Tuesday	4.	5	4-	Evening.
Wednesday	5. S.	5	o	Evening.
Thursday	6. S.	5-		
	E.		4 ᴜ	
Friday	7. S.	6 ᴜ	5	
Saturday	8. S. W. & E.	5-	5	
Sunday	9. N.	5-		
			2	
Monday	10. E. & N. E.	4-		
	N.	4 ᴜ	2	

May	11	The fame, ftorm and cold weather; in the evening a high and nipping wind, and in the night a fharp froft. The water froze in the kitchen, and an inch thick in the well.
Wednefday	12	For the moft part clear with lefs wind, but ftill cold; a great halo was feen round the fun, and the wind was high in the evening, but ceafed towards night, during which there was a froft.
Thurfday	13	Clear, windy and cold, with a froft in the night.
Friday	14	Clear, with a high wind and cold air; and in the night a pretty fharp froft.
Saturday	15	Between whiles clear, with a high wind and froft; in the night the water froze an inch thick.
Sunday	16	For the moft part clear, with a high wind and fharp froft; and in the night a froft.
Monday	17	Clear and windy, with a little froft in the night.
Tuefday	18	Clear and calm, but in the night a froft.
Wednefday	19	Foggy, with a little wind, and in the night a froft.
Thurfday	20	Clear, windy and cold weather, with a froft in the night.
Friday	21	The fame.
Saturday	22	The fame.
		During thefe days a little wind in the day time, but calm in the evenings.
Sunday	23	Clear with a little wind; the evening calm, but in the night a froft.
Monday	24	Clear, warm weather, and pretty calm, towards evening quite calm, and in the night a froft.
Tuefday	25	Hazy and calm.
Wednefday	26	The fame, but the afternoon windy.
Thurfday	27	Hazy and windy.

	Wind.	Barom.	Ther. open air.	
May	11. N.	2-	o	3 o'clock, P. M.
	N. E.	1-	o	
Wednesday 12.	N. N. E.	28 o-	2	
		27 11-	3	
Thursday 13.	E. by N.	11-	3	
Friday 14.	N E.	11-	2 o	
Saturday 15.	N. N. E.	28 2 o	o	clock 11 P. M.
Sunday 16.	N. N.	3 o	o	clock 8 P. M.
Monday 17.	N. & N. E.	2-	1	fupra degel.
Tuesday 18.	N. E. & E.	2-	1-	
Wednesday 19.	N. E. & E.	2	2-	clock 11 P. M.
Thursday 20.	N. N. E.	4-	2	clock 10 P. M.
Friday 21.	N. & N. E.	4-	2-	clock 10 P. M.
Saturday 22.	N. & N. E.	4-	3-	clock 10 P. M.
Sunday 23.	N. W.	28 2-	2-	fupra degel. clock 10 P. M.
Monday 24.	N.	28 1		
	S. E.	28 o o	4 o	
Tuesday 25.	S. E.	27 11-	5-	clock 11 half P. M.
Wednesday 26.	S. E.	11		
		10	6	clock 11 P. M.
Thursday 27.	S. E.	10-	6	Midnight.

May

May	28	The fame; in the night rain.
Saturday	29	Hazy, fhowery and windy.
Sunday	30	The fame.
		The evening windy and fhowery.
Monday	31	Hazy and windy.
		The evening clear.
June	1	Hazy, windy and fhowery.
Wednefday	2	Hazy and windy.
		The evening very windy.
Thurfday	3	Hazy and windy :
		From noon the weather remained calm.
Friday	4	Clear and calm :
		Towards the evening hazy and a little wind.
Saturday	5	Hazy, with fome wind and fhowers.
Sunday	6	The fame, with more wind.
Monday	7	Between whiles clear and fomewhat calm.
Tuefday	8	For the moft part clear and calm.
Wednefday	9	Between whiles clear and hazy, with a little wind.
Thurfday	10	The fame.
Friday	11	The forenoon clear and calm; the afternoon and evening hazy, but fomewhat calm with rain.
Saturday	12	Hazy, calm and fhowery.
Sunday	13	The fame, but more wind.
Monday	14	Hazy, with a little wind.
Tuefday	15	Rain during the whole day, with a little wind; in the evening and night a very high wind.
Wednefday	16	Hazy and ftormy during the whole day and evening.
Thurfday	17	Hazy, with a great ftorm, and by intervals violent fhowers of rain; towards noon three or four claps of thunder, but not very loud in the S. E. and S. in the afternoon the wind not fo high, and no rain.
Friday	18	Hazy, and a high wind; in the afternoon lefs wind with a little rain.

1751.

	Wind.	Barom.	Ther. open air.	
May	28. S. E.	10-	7 ʊ	clock 11 P. M.
Saturday	29. S.	8-	6	clock 11 P. M.
Sunday	30. S. & S. W.	9-		
	W. S. W.	28 2	6-	clock 10 P. M.
Monday	31. S.	4		
	S. to E.	5-	6-	clock 10 P. M.
June.	1. S. S. E.	4	8	clock 10 P. M.
Wednesday	2. S. S. E.	3 ʊ		
			8-	clock 10 P. M.
Thursday	3. S.	3		
		4	8-	clock 10 P. M.
		4	14	clock 2 P. M.
Friday	4. S. E.		8 ʊ	clock 11 P. M.
Saturday	5. S. S. E.	2	8	clock 10 P. M.
Sunday	6. S. & S. W.	27 9-	6	clock 10 half P. M.
Monday	7. W.	11	5.	clock 10 half P. M.
Tuesday	8. S. & S. E.	28 0 ʊ	5-	clock 11 P. M.
Wednesday	9. S. E.	27 9	8-	clock 10 P. M.
Thursday	10. N. E. & E.	6-	7-	clock 10 half P. M.
Friday	11. S. E.	7	13	clock 2 P. M.
	N. & S. W.	8	8-	clock 10 half P. M.
Saturday	12. S.	7-	8	clock 10 half P. M.
Sunday	13. S. E.	7-	8	clock 10 half P. M.
Monday	14. S. S. E.	10	8	clock 11 P. M.
Tuesday	15. S. E. & E.	27 11-		
	S. E.		9-	clock 11 half P. M.
Wednesday	16. S. E.	28 0-	10	clock 10 half P. M.
Thursday	17. S. S. E.	3	9	clock 11 P. M.
Friday	18. S. S. E.	5	9	clock 11 P. M.

1751.		The weather.
June	19	Hazy with fome wind ; the afternoon and evening calm.
Sunday	20	Hazy, rainy, and for the moft part calm ; in the afternoon clear, with a little wind.
Monday	21	Hazy and rainy, with fome wind.
Tuefday	22	Hazy, pretty windy, and rainy.
Wednefday	23	The fame ; in the evening rain and wind, and in the night ftorms and fnow in the mountains.
Thurfday	24	Hazy and cold weather, with a very high wind ; the evening clear, but the wind not fo high.
July	22	The forenoon clear, but the afternoon hazy.
	30	The weather for the moft part clear and warm.

	Wind.	Barom.		Ther. open air.
June	19 S.		5	9-	clock 11 P. M.
Sunday	20. S.				
	S. E.		4-	9	clock 11 P. M.
Monday	21. S. & S. W.		3	8	clock 10 half P. M.
Tuesday	22. S. to E. & S. W.		0-	8	clock 10 half P. M.
Wednesday	23. S. W.	27	10-		
	N.		9	6-	clock 10 P. M.
	N.				
Thursday	24. N.	28	0-	6-	clock 10 A. M.
	N.		1-	6	clock 10 P. M.
July	22. N. & S. E.	27	9	16	clock 1 P. M.
	30. N. & S. E.		11	17	clock 1 P. M.

REMARKS

REMARKS

ON THE

METEOROLOGICAL OBSERVATIONS.

THE barometer I made thefe obfervations by, was a *barometre ordinaire*, on which the divifions were meafured by French inches and lines.

The thermometer was conftructed with quick-filver, to prevent its receiving damage, if the cold fhould be very fevere. The divifions were according to Monfieur Reaumur's *thermometre*, that is, with eighty divifions or degrees between *frigus artificiale*, and that point where the fpirits or quick-filver rifes in boiling hot fpirits of wine, and ninety-five degrees between *frigus artificiale*, and that point to which the fpirits of wine rife in boiling hot fpirits, when the thermometer is fealed.

From the beginning of my obfervations, down to the firft of October 1750, they were made in a room where no warmth or heat could come, and the thermometer was hung out of the reach of the fun, which fcarce ever fhone in the room. Since that time I hung the thermometer in the open air, but not in the leaft expofed to the fun, and fo noted the greateft heat or cold, as appears by the column of the thermometer. It was this laft way that fome of the obfervations were made the firft year, which I have taken notice of in their proper place; and my remarks both on the barometer and thermometer, were according to that time of the day, when they were either higheft or loweft with the common fign, a half, a quarter, or an ovix.

Having defcribed the inftruments, and my manner of making thefe obfervations, it will not be amifs to collect in a fhort compafs, or to form a fummary of them, with regard to the heat, cold, and denfity of the air in Iceland, as it may be compared with the fame in Denmark..

According to my obfervations, the thermometer in the winter of 1749, did not fink lower than feven or eight degrees *infra degelationem*.

lationem. This happened on the 10th of March 1750, and was no very great froft, when one confiders that there are frofts commonly at Copenhagen, which fink the thermometer three or four degrees ftill lower. The thermometer was in Iceland 11 degrees *infra delegationem.* In the winter of 1750, which was feverer than the foregoing, and was even reckoned a fevere one by the Icelanders. The mercury in the thermometer funk 13 degrees the 25th of January 1751, at four o'clock, P. M. which is more than it commonly does at Copenhagen, though it has been ftill lower; for in 1709, it funk 16 degrees, and in February 1740, upwards of 18.

Upon the whole, it evidently appears from the obfervations, that the winters are not immoderately cold in Iceland, no frofts of any long duration having happened, but froft and thaw continually fucceeding each other as at Copenhagen; fo that the material difference of the winter muft confift in the length; becaufe in Iceland it feems to laft longer, as may be feen by the obfervations for both 1750, and 1751, in the former of which the froft lafted till the middle of April, and in the latter, till the middle of May, ice being even found an inch thick in the night of the 15th of May, and the frofts continuing in the nights till the 23d. It is likewife obfervable, that the month of May was in 1751, very cold in Denmark, but not fo cold as in Iceland.

From cold, it will not be improper to animadvert on the heat. In Auguft 1749, the thermometer rofe 13 degrees *fupra degelationem:* in July 1750, it likewife rofe 13 degrees; and on the 30th of June in 1751, it rofe 17, which laft is its ufual complement of rifing at Copenhagen, whereby it may be feen, as one would naturally expect, that the fummers are not fo hot as in Denmark, though the difference is not fo great as many perhaps imagine. It is remarkable, that the fummer of 1750, the hotteft ever known in Denmark, was very moderate in Iceland; for towards the latter end of July, when the thermometer rofe at Copenhagen 25½ degrees, it did not rife higher than 10 or 11 in Iceland. Thus heat and cold cannot be deemed as correfponding to the fame degrees in both places.

G g g

When

When it was but moderately hot at Copenhagen in 1751, the thermometer rose higher in Iceland than it did the two preceding summers, and one may also see by these observations, that the air in Iceland is not subject to great changes in respect to heat and cold as in Denmark, and therefore according to the rules or opinions of the learned in physicks, the climate must be more healthy, daily experience convincing us, that weak and tender people in other countries are affected by any unusual great degree of heat or cold. As for the climate of Iceland, it agreed extremely well with me, and I found it much more agreeable than I expected, or had any idea of; because at Copenhagen it is generally compared with that of Greenland, whereas it rather should with that of Denmark or Norway.

Though the air is subject to few changes in regard to heat and cold, yet its density or weight is pretty considerable. The weight of the air most commonly at Copenhagen, according to barometrical observations, is computed at twenty-eight inches of quick-silver in the barometer. Sometimes it rises a few lines higher, and sometimes sinks a few lower; but the whole difference, taking one time with another, does not amount to upwards of twelve lines or one inch. The barometer seldom sinks at Copenhagen to twenty-seven inches, and when it does, severe and stormy weather generally ensues, especially if it falls suddenly, and does not last long.

It is quite otherwise in Iceland; for on the 11th of January, 11th of February, and 24th of March, in 1750, the barometer stood at twenty-six inches, and four or five lines: on the 22d and 23d of November in 1749, the 5th and 6th of October, and 17th and 18th of November 1750, it stood at twenty-eight inches, and seven, eight, and nine lines higher; so that the difference between the highest and lowest, amounts to two inches and five lines, which is very considerable. I allow that the difference of the barometer at Copenhagen may exceed, though very rarely, twelve lines or one inch: but it is plain, that this great difference with density or weight of the air is frequent in Iceland, and it is even remarkable, that very often when the barometer has been high in Iceland, the weather was very bad, and *vice versâ*, very fine, when the barometer had been very low, which is quite the

reverse

reverfe of the rules hitherto eftablifhéd, with regard to the baro-meters rifing and falling. It was not poffible for me from thefe few obfervations, to fix the fpecific denfity or gravity of the air, refpectively to Denmark and Iceland, as fuch muft require many more years obfervations, though it feems to me upon an average, that the air in Denmark and Iceland is of the fame denfity, or equally ponderous.

The wind and weather in Iceland, are alfo much the fame as in Denmark; but it is not to be underftood, that the weather is alike at one and the fame time, which cannot be expected in two countries fo very remote from each other.

The north lights appear oftner in Iceland than in Denmark, and are not for the moft part fucceeded by bad weather; they make the nights much lighter, and are very convenient to tra-vellers, or thofe who have any thing to do in the open air.

Fogs feldom happen in Iceland, which is quite the contrary of what Mr. Anderfon afferts in his treatife of this country, wherein he has taken a deal of pains without any juft reafon, to paint it in the blackeft colours.

F I N I S.

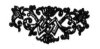

CPSIA information can be obtained at www.ICGtesting.com
Printed in the USA
BVOW06*2016010216

434434BV00026B/130/P

9 781296 568764